Quick Reference Atlas of Dermatology

Dr Vivienne Owen Ankrett
MB. BCh. MRCGP. DRCOG

Dr Ian Williams
MB. BCh. MRCGP. DRCOG

Dedication

We should like to dedicate this book to each other for a truly joint venture.

Thanks also to our children David & Kirsty who once again have been very patient during its preparation.

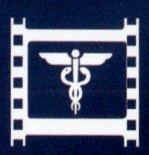

M.S.L.
MEDICAL SLIDE LIBRARY

Published by MSL, 33 Dornden Drive, Langton Green,
Tunbridge Wells, Kent, England UK TN3 0AE

Copies available direct from publisher

ISBN: 0 9535982 0 9

Typeset & Printed by Media-Flo, Langton Green,
Tunbridge Wells, Kent, England, UK TN3 0EG

©1999 All world-wide rights reserved. No part of this publication may be produced, copied, stored in a retrieval system or transmitted in any form or by any means, without prior permission of the copyright holder.

Author's Disclaimer: The authors would like to emphasise that the content of this book is based upon current medical practice and common therapeutic options at the time of writing. Medical science however is constantly changing and readers are encouraged to remain abreast of developments. The authors have endeavoured to compile accurate and complete information to the best of their knowledge. They are not however responsible for any errors or the consequences of using this information.

Special thanks to Merit Publishing International, 1st Floor, 35 Winchester Street, Basingstoke, Hampshire RG21 7EE, England & 8260 NW 49th Manor, Coral Springs, Florida 33067, USA for publishing our first book "Atlas Casebook of Primary Care" 1999 ISBN: 1 873413 56 4 in which several of the illustrations contained within this book also appear.

Introduction

This book represents our second sortie into medical publishing.
Our first publication " Atlas Casebook of Primary Care" Merit Publishing International 1999, dealt with 100 conditions seen by us in primary care and presented in an easy to read quiz form.

On this occasion we have focused upon dermatological conditions and manifestations of disease commonly encountered by the physician, primary or secondary. The "bullet point" format has been adopted for ease of reading and learning. We have endeavoured to address the most relevant and important facts pertinent to daily practice. The information is, therefore, not all encompassing. The finer histopathology, immunology or hospital based diagnostic techniques have not been included for the sake of brevity and practical interest.

We hope to illustrate how vital a working knowledge of dermatology is to the practitioner yet it is an area that is often very briefly visited in medical school teaching. There is nothing that can substitute for experience but these photographs illustrate the wide and varied range of conditions that can be encountered in primary care.

The Authors

Ian Williams and Vivienne Owen Ankrett are husband and wife and general practitioners based in Tunbridge Wells, Kent and Crowborough, East Sussex, England.

As well as being primary care physicians, they have been taking medical photographs for the past seventeen years and have created MSL - the "Medical Slide Library".

They regularly supply illustrations and articles for both the medical press as well as international publishing companies.

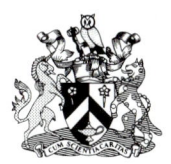

They are three times winners of the Royal College of General Practitioners
Scottish Council / South East Scotland Faculty
Ian Stokoe Memorial Award
For:
"Original work produced in the context of primary care
with specific emphasis on the quality of illustrations"

ABSCESS

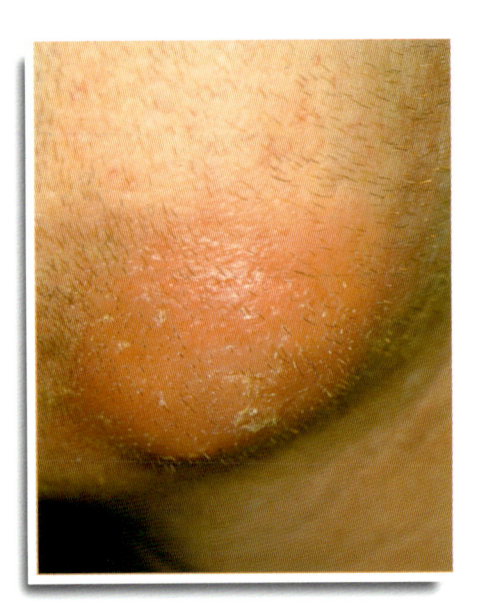

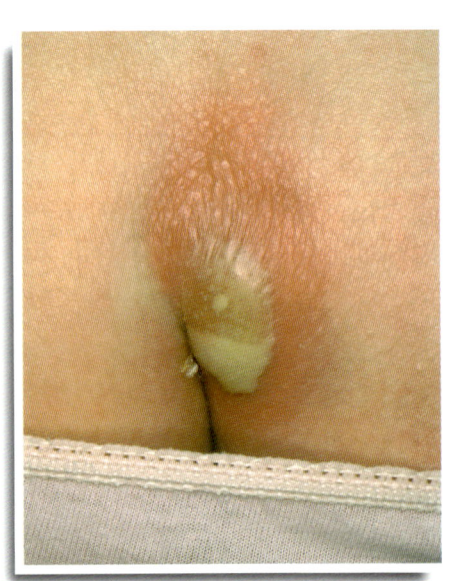

- Circumscribed collection of pus
- Acute / chronic localised infection (central fluctuance when established)
- Associated tissue destruction
- Children, teenagers + young adults, Male > Female
- Staphylococcus aureus or sterile
- Predisposing factors: chronic Staph' carrier, diabetes, poor hygiene + immune deficiencies
- Treatment: incision + drainage. If symptomatic - antibiotics e.g. Flucloxacillin
- Treat proven Staph' carrier site - topical antibiotic e.g. Fusidic acid or Mupirocin

ACANTHOSIS NIGRICANS

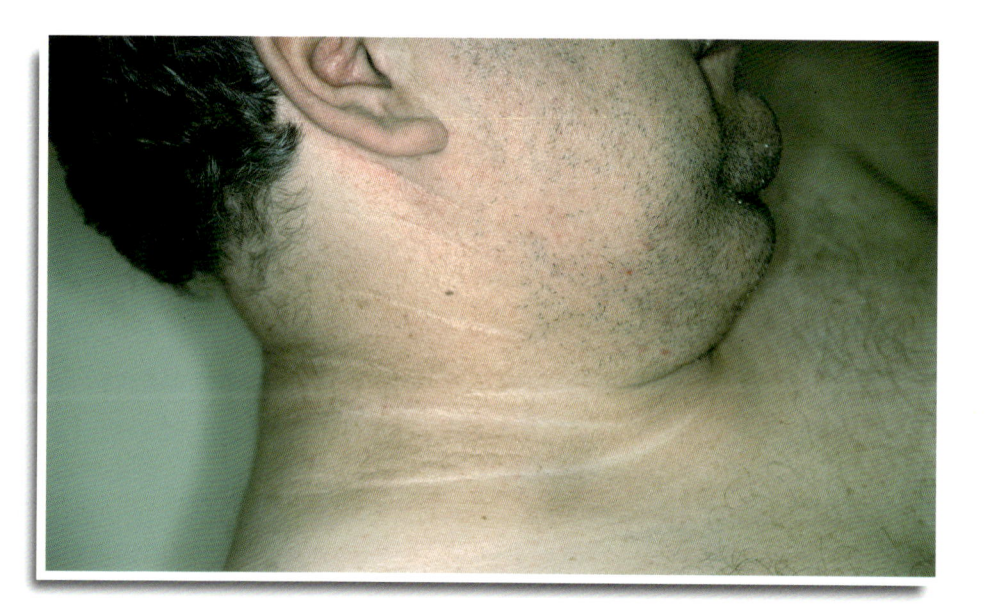

- Rare epidermal disorder with hyperkeratosis + hyperpigmentation
- Velvety thickening / wartiness of skin of dorsa hands, axillae, neck, elbows, nipples + umbilicus
- Dark brown pigmentation of major flexures with ↑ skin markings + skin tags
- 5 recognised types - all insidious onset
    1. Pseudo acanthosis nigricans associated with obesity + insulin resistance
    2. Associated with diabetes + acromegaly
    3. Familial benign juvenile type - dominantly inherited + regresses with age
    4. Drug induced - Oral contraceptives, Nicotinic acid + Stilboestrol
    5. Associated with primary abdominal cavity malignancy (adenocarcinomas) >40 years old, palmar skin + buccal mucosa thickening
- Treatment: ↓ weight, exclude endocrine disorder, stop causative drug + exclude carcinoma
- Acanthosis can proceed other symptoms of malignancy by up to 5 years
- Removal of tumour → regression of acanthosis

quick reference atlas of dermatology

ACNE ROSACEA

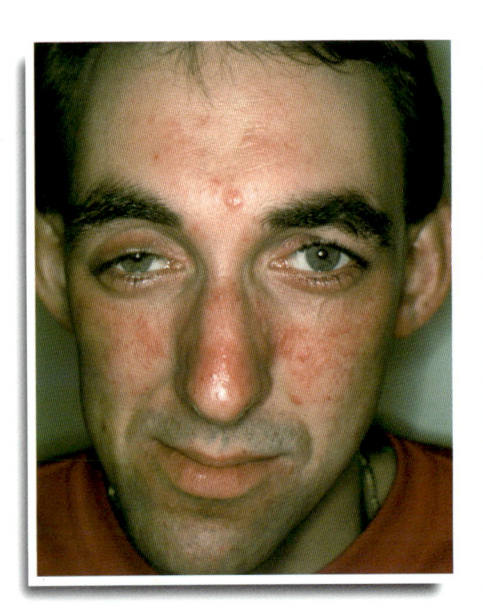

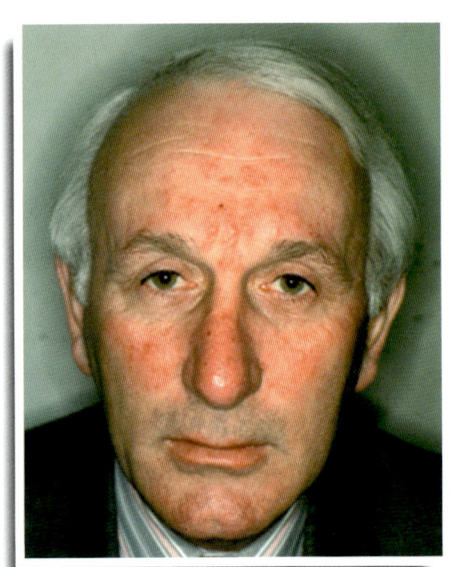

- Inflammatory disorder of face - cause unknown
- Peak incidence 4th + 5th decade, Female > Male, Celtic races
- Persistent erythema of cheeks +/- forehead, nose + chin
- Non tender papules, telangiectasia + oedema
- Cysts + scarring do not occur,
- Rapid response to oral antibiotics e.g. Tetracyclines or topical Metronidazole
- If severe - low dose isotretinoin. Erythema can persist despite therapy
- Worsened by stress, alcohol + hot beverages
- Course is prolonged, frequent recurrences, disappears spontaneously after several years
- Complications - blepharitis, keratitis (+ corneal ulcers), rhinophyma Male > Female
- Topical steroids can induce rosacea-like rash (steroid rosacea)

ACNE VULGARIS

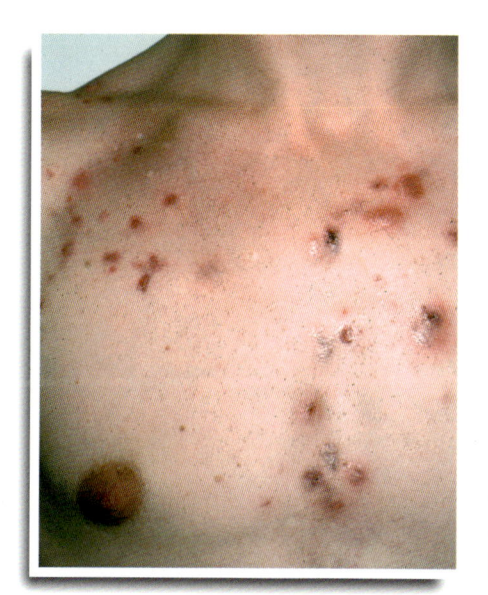

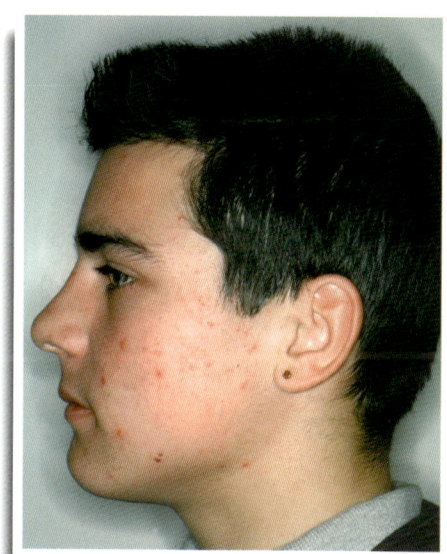

- Disease of sebaceous follicles,
- Hallmark is a comedone, closed (whitehead) or open (blackhead) - colour due to melanin
- Primarily Caucasians, peak incidence 13 - 16 years (range 8 - 40)
- Occurs earlier in Females but Males more severely affected
- Primary sites : face (often associated with seborrhoea), chest + back
- Genetic factors determine clinical pattern + severity (severe in XYY)
- No dietary influences proven. Stress, premenstruum, Autumn / Winter - aggravating factors
- Tender papules / pustules / nodules / cysts + sinus tracts
- Ice pick or papular scarring

quick reference atlas of dermatology

ACNE VULGARIS

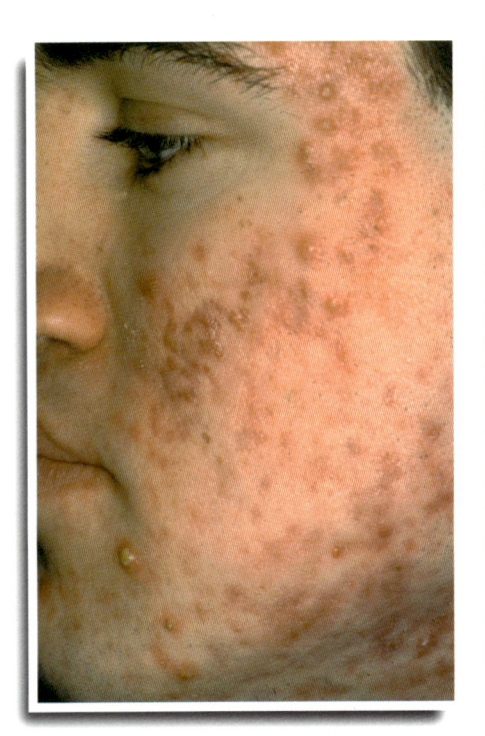

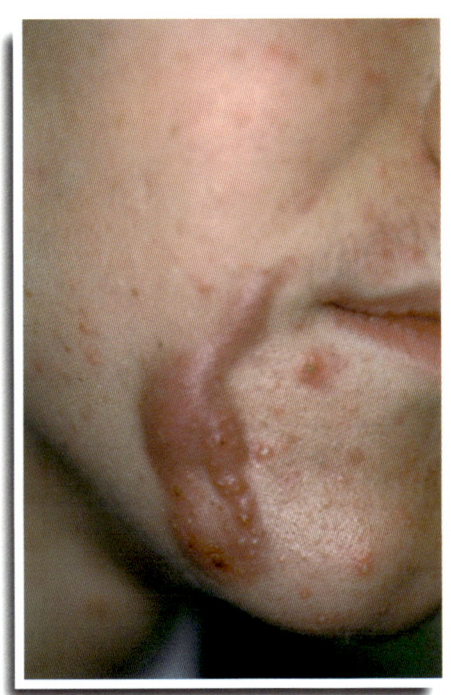

- Treatment depends on predominant lesions, often combination therapy needed
- Comedones - keratolytic agents
- Inflammatory lesions - long term antibiotics (topical or oral), anti-androgens in women
- Cystic acne - Isotretinoin
- Sunlight may help

ALOPECIA AREATA

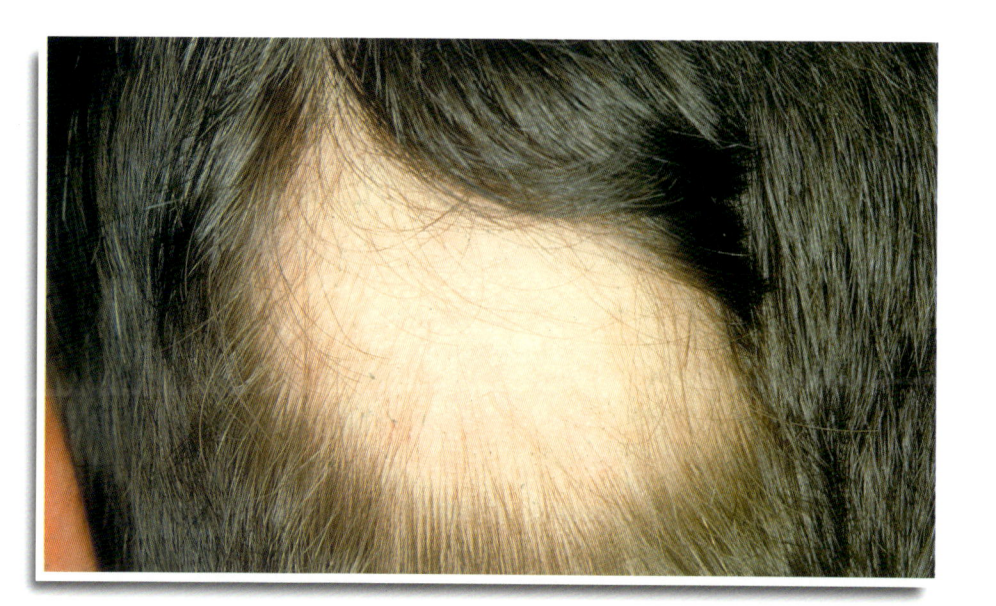

- Cessation of hair growth in well demarcated areas of scalp
- No associated redness / scaling of scalp
- Primarily children + young adults, Male = Female
- Exclamation mark-like hair stumps visible in affected area
- Primarily scalp (+ beard area in males)
- Only pigmented hairs affected + subsequently lost
- Several areas may appear → coalesce (poor prognostic sign if on occiput)
- If atopic individual - outcome less encouraging
- Recovery spontaneous but unpredictable, most recover after 3 - 6 months
- New hair initially white then darkens
- Associated finding - dystrophic "hammered brass" nails

ALOPECIA TOTALIS

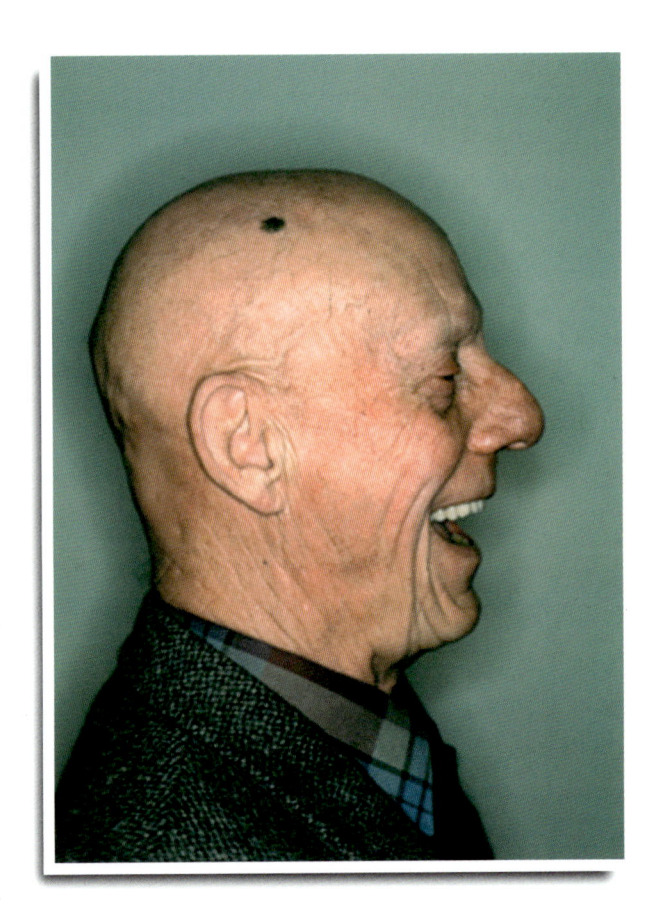

- All hair lost from scalp + eyebrows
- Affects all races
- Alopecia universalis - all body hair lost
- Autoimmune - sometimes associated with thyroid disease
- Total alopecia pre-puberty - poor prognosis
- Treatment: oral steroids often used for up to a month
- Psychological support very important
- Outcome unpredictable - a third of patients never have hair regrowth

ANGIO-OEDEMA

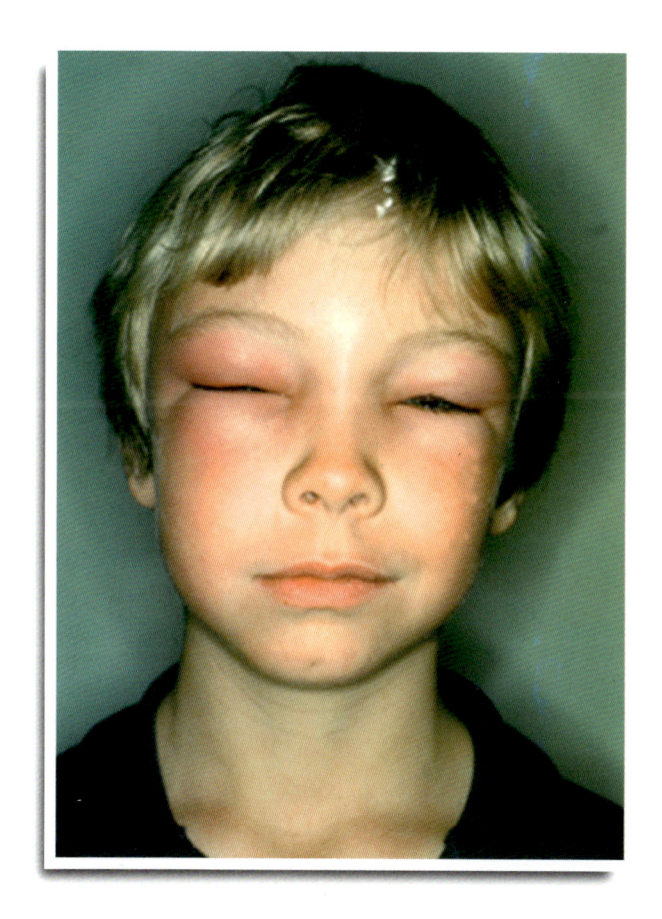

- Urticaria affecting lips, tongue + eyelids (swelling of deep dermal + subcutaneous tissue)
- More severe immediate hypersensitivity reaction
- Typical response to food stuffs or drugs
- Occurs in 1: 10,000 courses of Penicillin → resulting in death in 1-5 : 100,000 courses
- Severe systemic signs - wheezing, oral swelling, vomiting, abdo' pain, diarrhoea or hypotensive collapse
- Usually resolves within 24 - 48 hours
- Treatment: antihistamines +/- H2 antagonists, steroids
- Severe reaction - I.M. Adrenaline dose according to age / body weight

ANGIOMA - CHERRY
"Campbell De Morgan Spot"

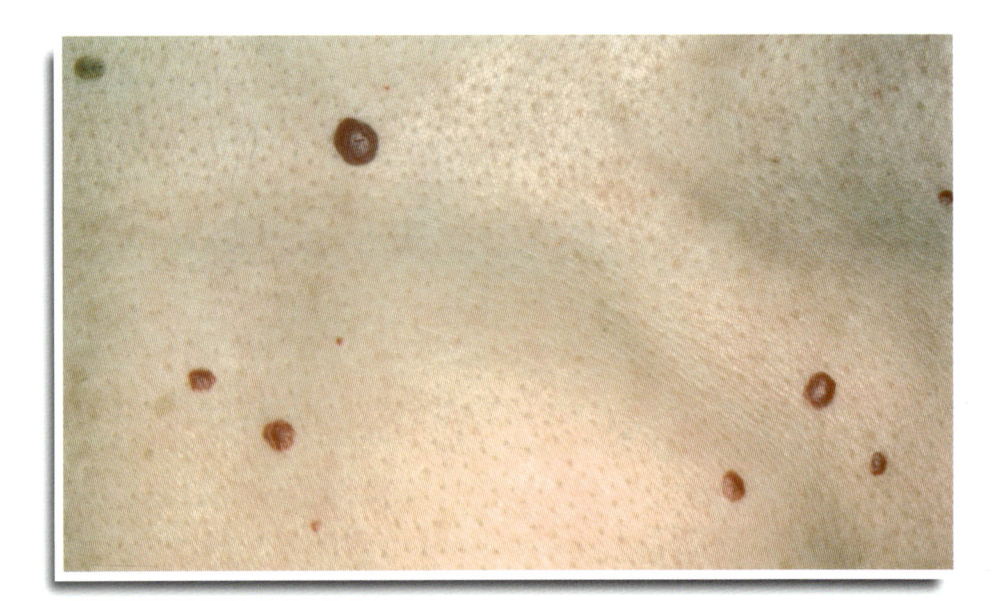

- 1 - 4 mm bright red / purple papules on trunk + proximal limbs
- Occurs over 35 years of age and is a harmless condition
- Treatment: electro or laser coagulation if small, formal excision if large
- Cryosurgery not effective

BASAL CELL CARCINOMA
"BCC or Rodent Ulcer"

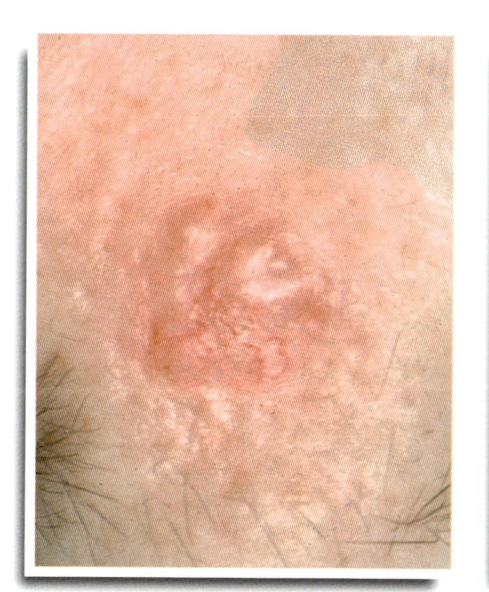

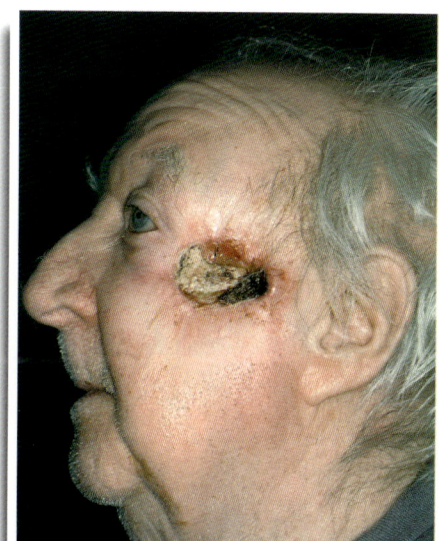

- Commonest malignant tumour of skin, slow growing + locally invasive
- Male > Female, usually after age 40
- Usually single (can be multiple), primarily on face (can occur anywhere)
- Primarily flat scaling macule / plaque or pearly nodule
- Flecks of or uniformly pigmented, dilated blood vessels on surface
- Larger lesions hard + firm with raised rolled edges, may ulcerate
- Invades deeply at nasolabial folds, ear canal, canthi + posterior auricular sulcus
- Predisposing factors: red hair, blue eyes, freckles, previous X rays for acne
- Treatment: local excision or radiotherapy → 95% cure, cryotherapy → 70% cure
- Prevention: high protection sun screen

quick reference atlas of dermatology

BECKER'S NAEVUS

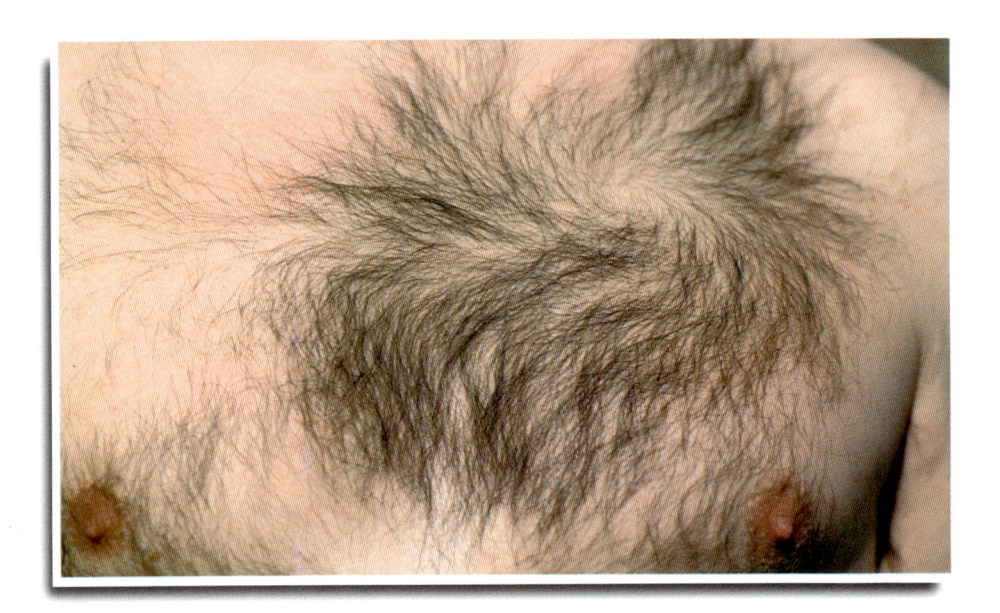

- Common acquired, benign, pigmented hamartoma of epidermis + hair follicles
- Male > Female, develops in adolescence
- Large, pigmented area with hypertrichosis (coarse dark hairs)
- Primarily shoulder + upper chest (5:1)
- Permanent, becomes wartier with time, not pre-malignant
- Associations (rare): hypoplasia of arm or breast
- Treatment: excision usually impractical, depilation helpful cosmetically
- Q switched ruby laser can ablate pigmentation

BLACKHEADS
"Comedones"

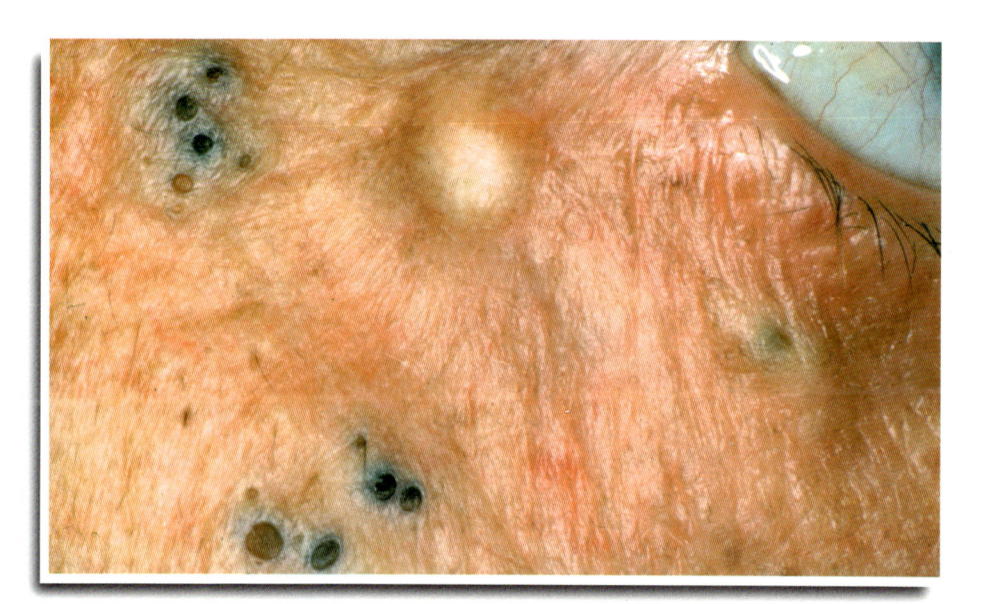

- Sebaceous follicle containing altered sebum + cellular debris
- Black colouration due to melanin
- Closed comedone = whitehead with no punctum
- Open comedone = blackhead
- Hallmark of acne
- Associated with solar elastosis around eyes of elderly
- Treatment: comedone extraction if few lesions present
- Gentle exposure to sun light
- Keratolytic agents to remove keratin plug + open follicle
- Resistant closed comedones - cautery after use of EMLA under occlusion (Dermatologist)

quick reference atlas of dermatology

BLUE NAEVUS
"Blue Neuro Naevus"

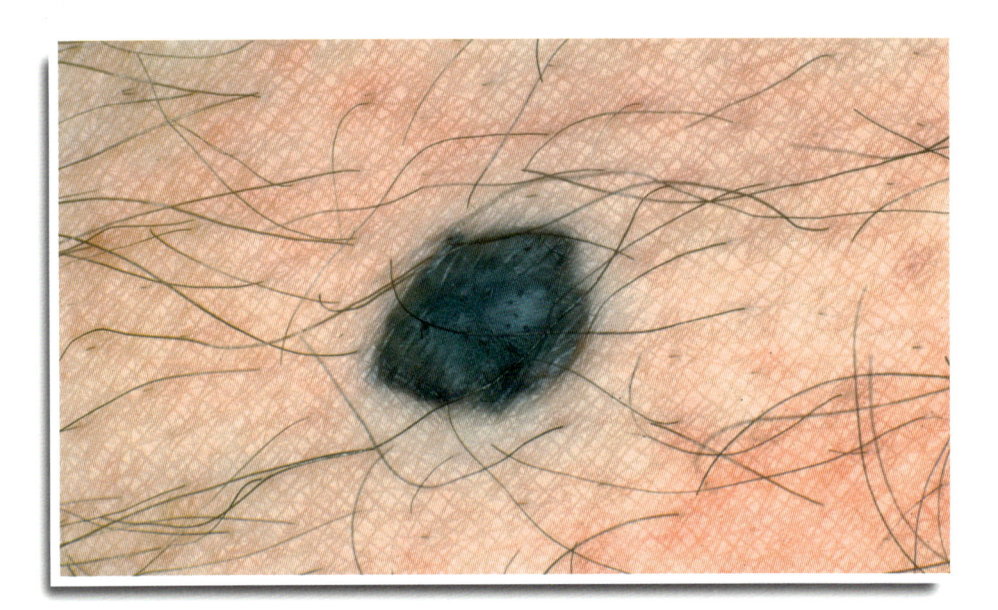

- Male = Female, any age
- Acquired naevus
- Melanocytes deep in dermis appear blue / black due to Tindel's effect
- Small, regular, smooth, slightly raised + remain unchanged
- Primarily dorsum hands + feet, buttocks + face
- Treatment: not usually required
- Excise for cosmetic reasons. Warning - anterior chest wall scars often unsightly

BOWEN'S DISEASE

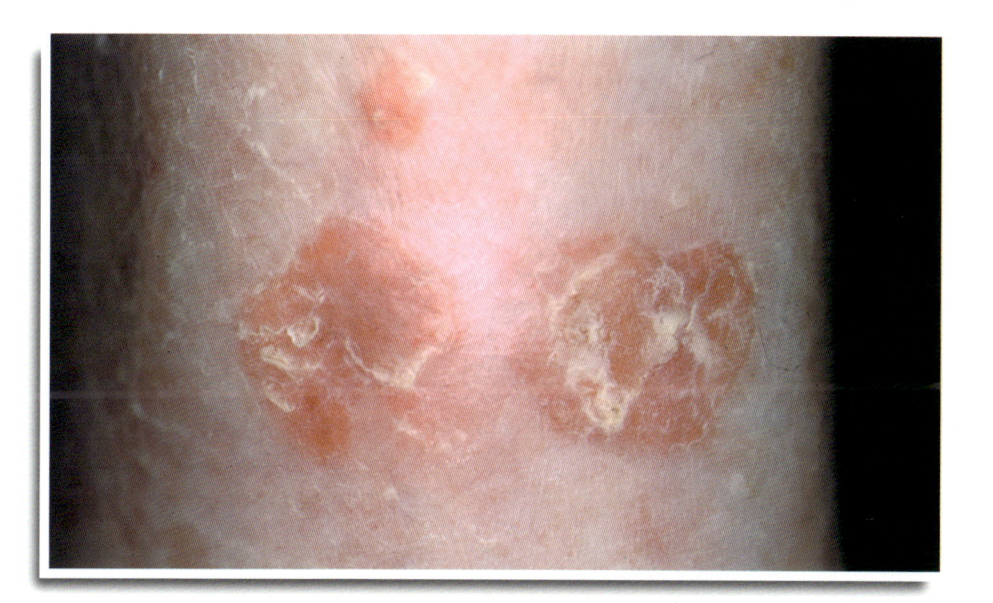

- Intraepidermal epithelioma (form of SCC in situ)
- Well defined, slow growing, red scaling plaque, often solitary
- On sun exposed skin (often front of lower legs in middle aged / elderly female)
- Resistant to therapy e.g. topical steroids + emollients
- Treatment: curettage + cautery, cryotherapy, local excision or radiotherapy
- Site of lesion dictates approach (care not to produce ulcer by excising lower leg lesions)
- If on unexposed skin consider arsenic as a cause

CAFÉ AU LAIT

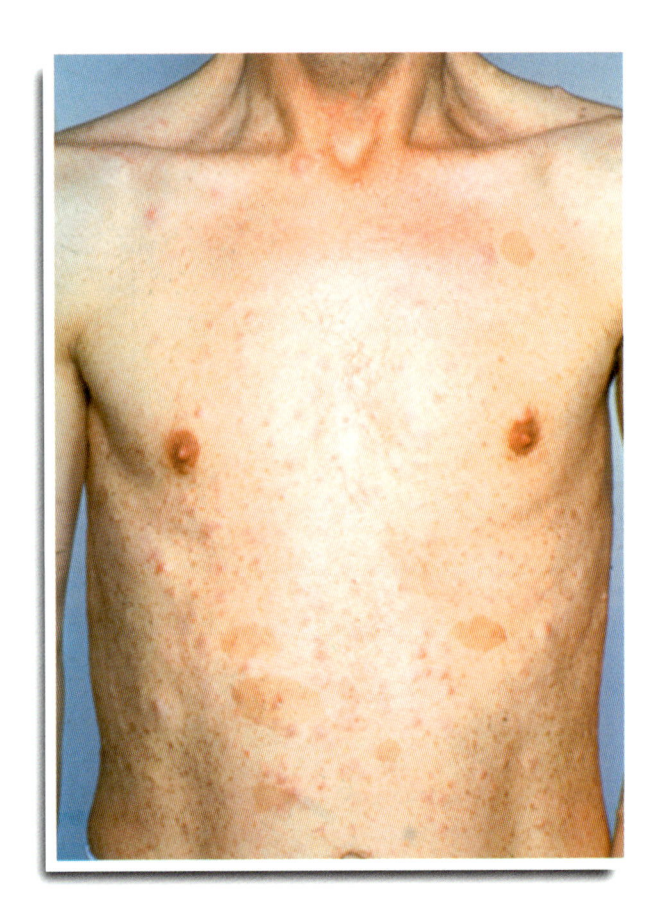

- Solitary lightly pigmented patch - can be seen in normal individuals
- Light brown, round / oval, 2 - 10 cm diameter
- Occur at birth / early childhood (under 5 years)
- > 6 lesions - neurofibromatosis likely (Von Recklinghausen's disease):
- Inherited neurocutaneous disorder
- Autosomal dominant with variable penetrance (some spontaneous mutations)
- If child reaches 5 years old without lesions - not affected
- Prenatal diagnosis available
- Genetic counselling for affected families

CANDIDA
"Moniliasis"

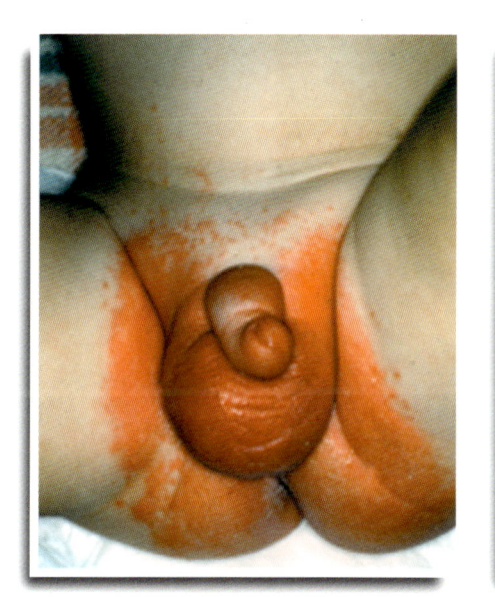

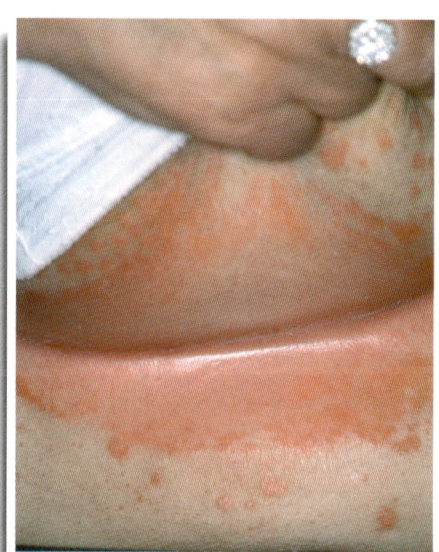

- Latin : candidus = white
- Superficial fungal infection occurring at warm moist sites
- Male = Female, all ages. In infants affects napkin area + mouth
- Causative agents: primarily candida albicans endogenous to oropharynx + GI tract
- Napkin dermatitis → can represent primary or secondary infection
- Bright red erythema + oedema with papular / pustular lesions
- Involves creases / flexures, marginal scaling + "satellite spots". Confluent lesions → erosions
- Treatment: primary prevention with attention to hygiene + leave area exposed when possible
- Topical antifungal + barrier creams

CANDIDA - ORAL

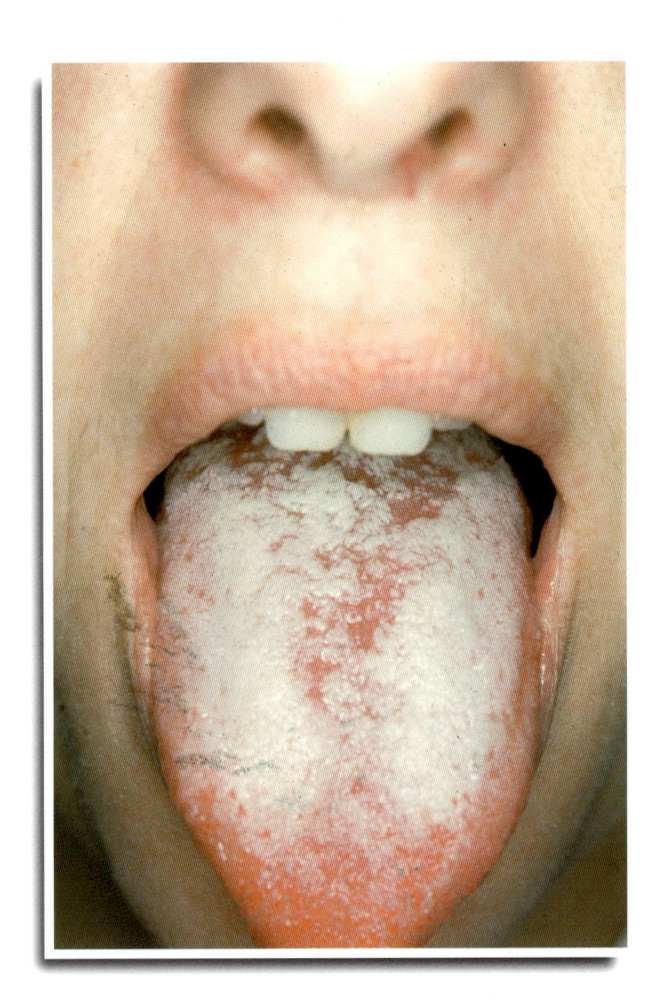

- 60 - 80% of oral infections due to candida albicans
- Normal commensal (mouth + gut) in 30% population.
- In neonates usually acquired from maternal genital tract at birth
- 1-2 mm white pustules → plaques on dorsum tongue, buccal mucosa + palate
- Easily scraped off to reveal red base
- Can involve oesophagus → dysphagia. Severe if immuno-compromised patient
- Treatment: oral suspensions + gels, systemic antifungals if severe
- Dental plates / dummies important source of reinfection.

CAPILLARY HAEMANGIOMA
"Strawberry Naevus"

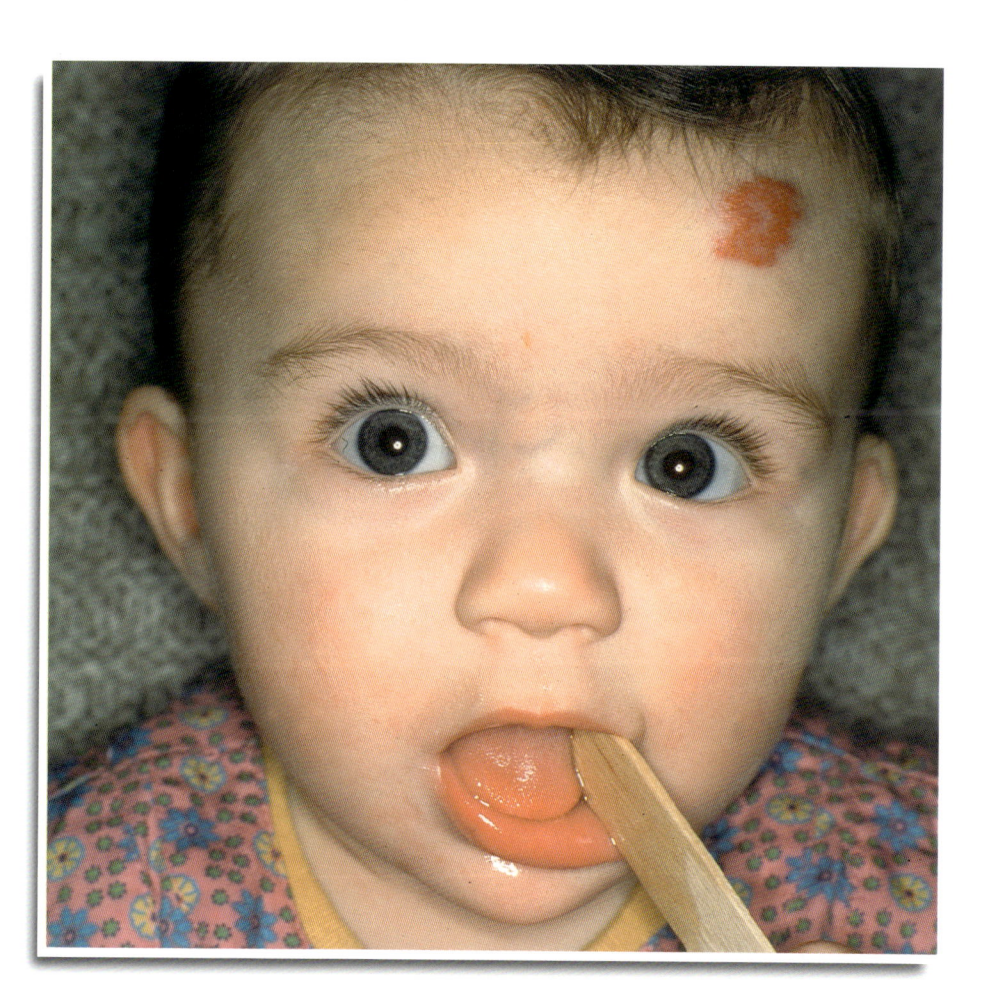

- Benign developmental defect of capillaries, superficial + deep components
- 1 - 2% Caucasians, more common in prem. / low birth weight babies
- Appear usually within 1st month of life as flat pink patch
- Rapid enlargement during 1st year + spontaneous regression usually by 7th year
- Single or multiple, soft rounded bright red nodules
- 50% on head / neck, 25% on trunk, also seen on napkin area
- Complications: bleeding + ulceration
- Treatment: reassurance + plastic surgery only if problematic

quick reference atlas of dermatology

CARBUNCLE

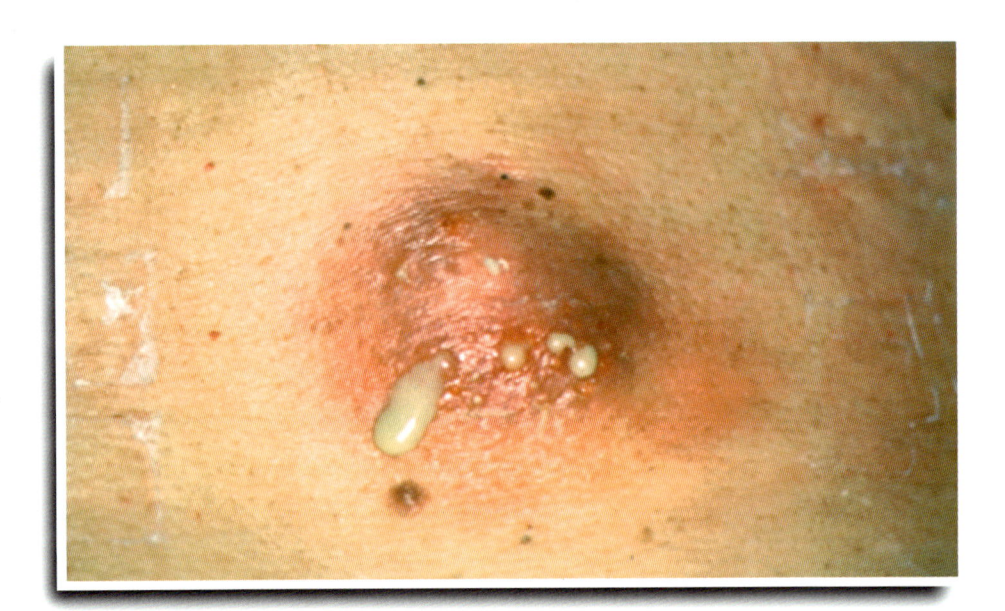

- Male > Female, children + young adults
- Indurated, painful nodule with punctum within dermis
- Interconnecting abscesses of several adjacent hair follicles
- Multiple sieve-like openings on surface
- Infection usually Staph' Aureus, patient often a carrier at other site e.g. nose or perineum
- Associated with diabetes, poor hygiene, obesity + debility
- Treatment: if pointing incision + drainage, otherwise oral antibiotics
- Folliculitis → Furuncles → Carbuncle - a continuum of severity of Staph' infection

quick reference atlas of dermatology

CELLULITIS

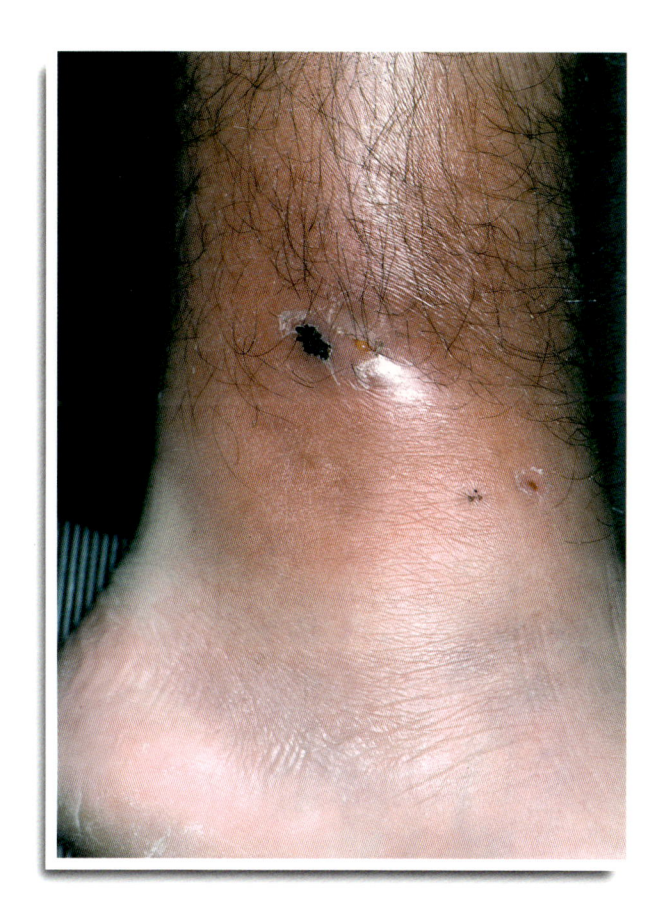

- Infection of lower dermis + subcutaneous tissues
- Group A, C or G Beta Haemolytic Streptococcus or Staph' Aureus
- Adults - Staph' or Strep'. Children <3 years - Staph', Haemophilus + Gp A Strep'
- Red, hot, tender area of skin - usually obvious source of infection e.g. leg ulcer, eczema
- Less well defined area of erythema than in erysipelas
- Can → Lymphangitis + lymphadenopathy, but no blistering or systemic effects
- Treatment: parenteral penicillin if severe, or oral for at least 2 weeks
- Exclude diabetes if slow to respond
- Risk factors: diabetes, malnutrition, immunosuppression, renal failure,
- Others include: drug + alcohol excess, carcinoma + lymphoedematous limb

quick reference atlas of dermatology

CHICKENPOX

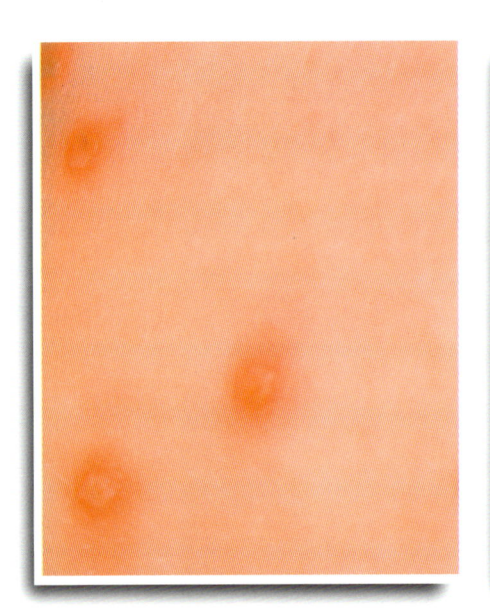

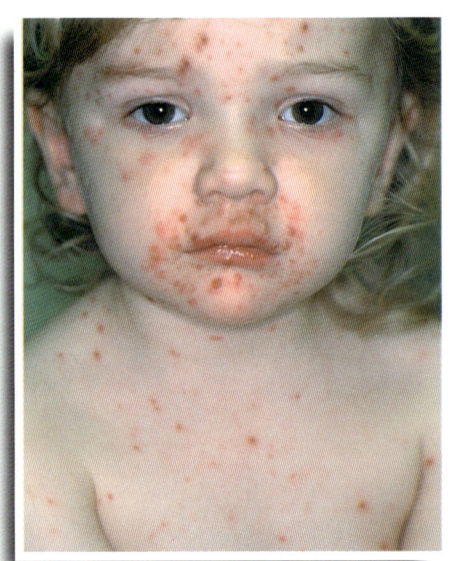

- DNA virus - Varicella Zoster, highly infectious
- Droplet transmission or contact with vesicle fluid, or patient with Herpes Zoster
- Incubation period 14 - 21 days, 1 -2 days prodromal malaise, fever + headache
- Erythematous papules → tense turbid vesicles (rim of erythema) → crusting + resolution
- Appear in crops over 4 -5 days, very itchy. Secondary infection → pock mark scars
- Complications: encephalitis, pneumonia (Staph'), recurrence as H. Zoster, Reye's Syndrome
- Treatment: conservative measures only, antiviral agent if severe or immuno-compromised
- Varicella Zoster Immuno Globulin to non immune pregnant women + vulnerable exposed patients
- Varicella Zoster virus vaccines for specific individuals

CHLOASMA
"Melasma"

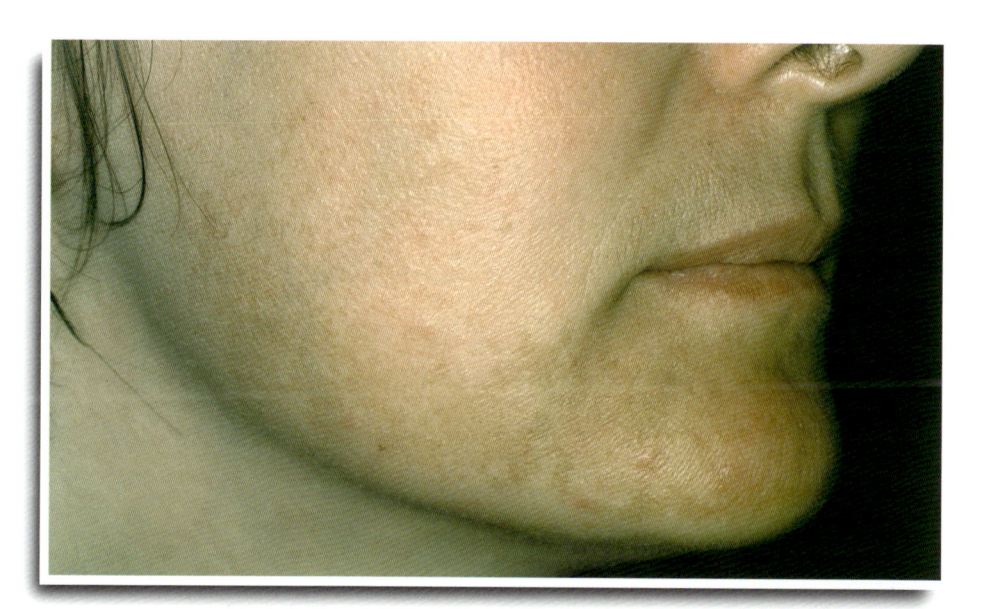

- Greek: Chloasma - green spot, Melasma - black spot
- Female (90%) >> Male (10%), dark skinned or black individuals, sunny climates
- Well defined, symmetrical patterned pigmentation affecting forehead, chin + cheeks
- Initially light brown - darkening with sun exposure or in premenstruum
- Seen as the "mask of pregnancy", with oral contraceptive use or idiopathic
- Treatment: unhelpful, sun screen can reduce pigmentation, reduces slowly after childbirth
- Retin A + Azelaic acid may help with months of treatment if patient very distressed
- Middle of abdomen darkening = linea nigra

CRADLE CAP

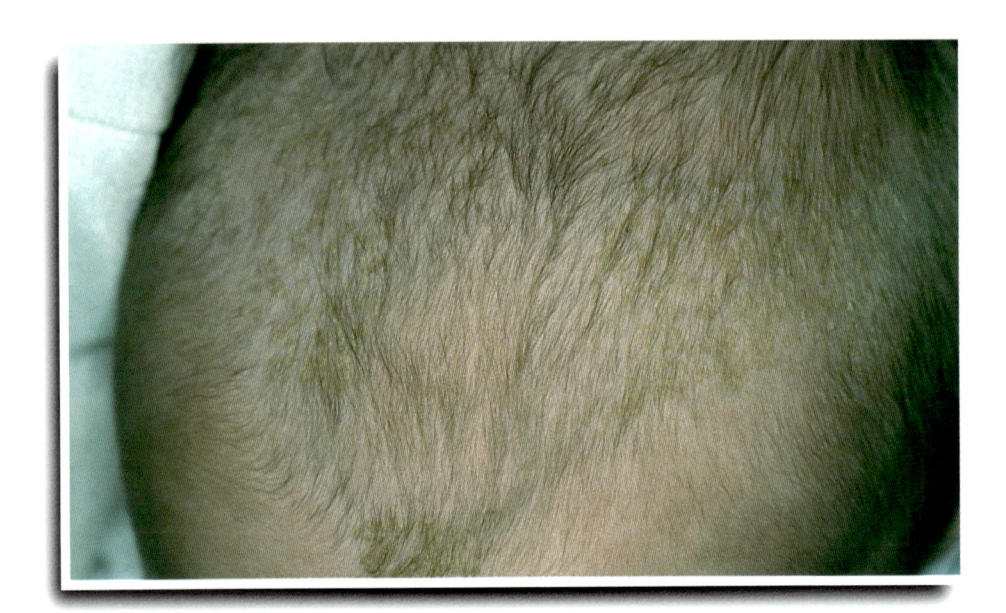

- Infantile seborrhoeic dermatitis affecting scalp
- Age 2 - 6 weeks, definitely within first 6 months
- Large yellow, greasy scales (desquamated skin cells) that crust scalp
- May progress to face, eyebrows, behind ears + napkin area
- Skin is red, moist + flakes at edges
- Treatment: mild shampoo 3-4 times a week, arachis, almond or olive oil massaged into scalp lifts scales
- Severe cases - weak corticosteroid lotions

quick reference atlas of dermatology

CYST OF MALHERBE

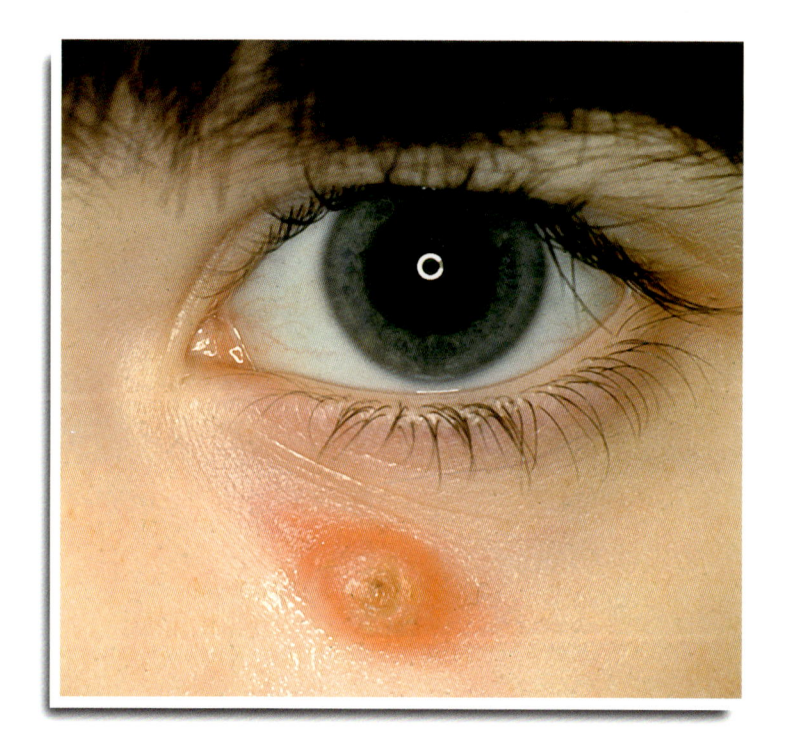

- Calcifying epithelioma / pilomatrixoma
- Hamartoma originating from hair follicle which frequently calcifies
- Commonest appendage tumour in childhood
- Hard, solitary, subcutaneous nodule primarily on face or upper body
- May attain considerable size
- Treatment: local excision

DERMATITIS - ARTEFACTA

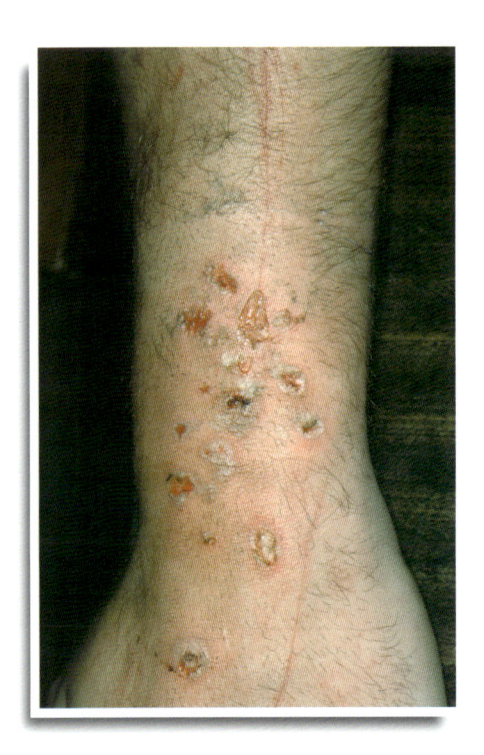

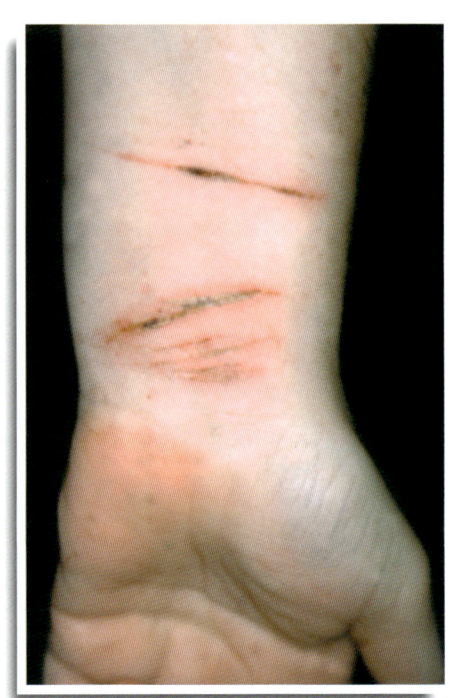

- Female >> Male, young + often paramedical
- Consider in any unexplained inflammatory rash or ulcer
- Burns, corrosive injuries, digging, picking, hair pulling + lichenification
- Clues - lesions have straight sides / lines rather than round / oval
- Occur only where patient can reach
- Underlying reason to be addressed (often psychiatric assessment / management)
- Direct confrontation / accusation of no help

DERMATITIS - CONTACT
"Exogenous Dermatitis"

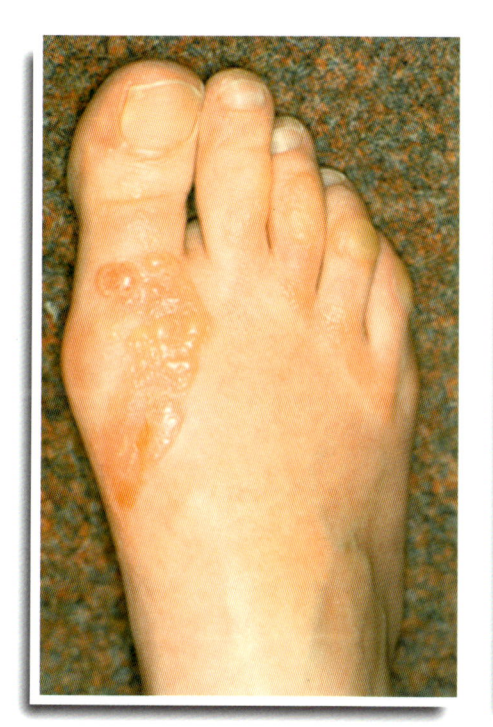

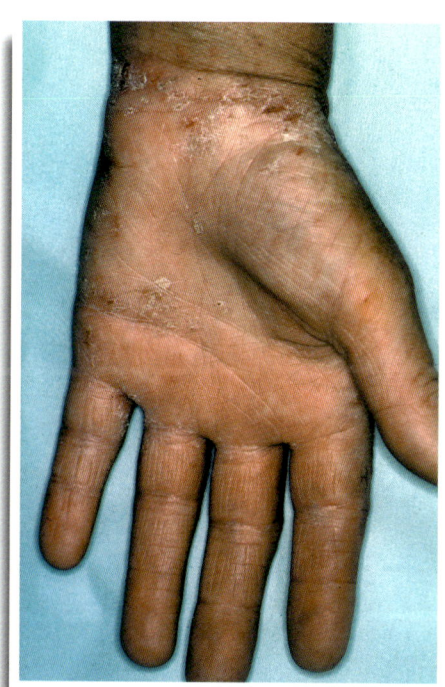

- Delayed / cell mediated, type IV hypersensitivity reaction
- Sensitisation persists indefinitely + desensitisation rarely possible
- Contact allergic (only sensitised patient) - at points of contact with sensitising material, rash can spread
- Contact irritant (anyone) - mainly hands ("housewife's dermatitis"), non allergic due to chemical irritant
- Skin reaction / changes the same whatever the cause (i.e. rashes look the same)
- Detailed occupational + domestic history vital, former important medico-legally
- Patch testing important
- Treatment: avoidance, protection + topical therapy (emollients + steroids)

DERMATITIS - LIP LICKING

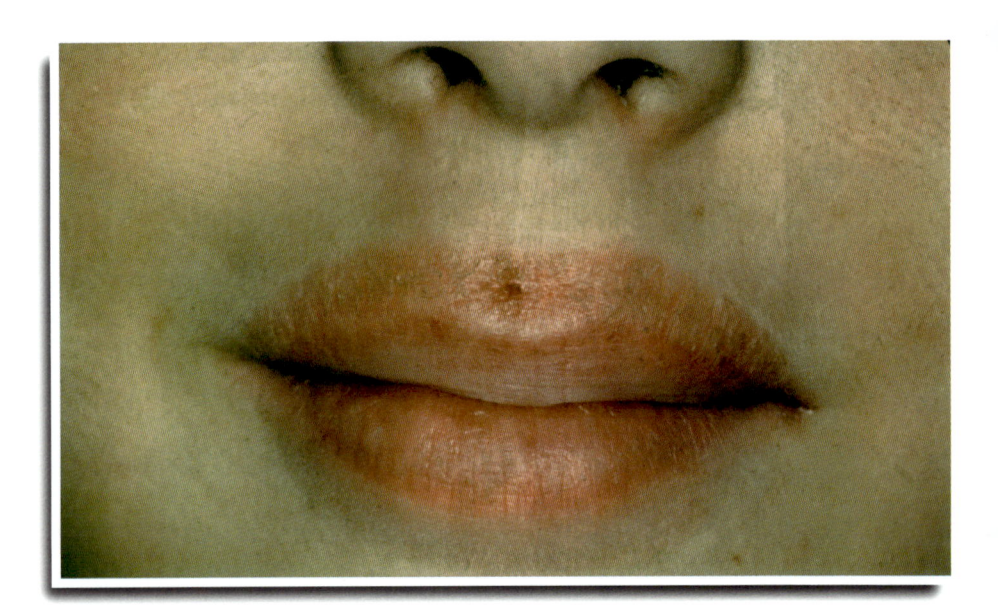

- Well defined, peri oral dermatitis due to habit tic
- Repetitive licking → irritation + chaffing
- Dry + scaling
- Treatment: discouragement of tic (difficult), barrier creams

DERMATITIS - PERIORAL

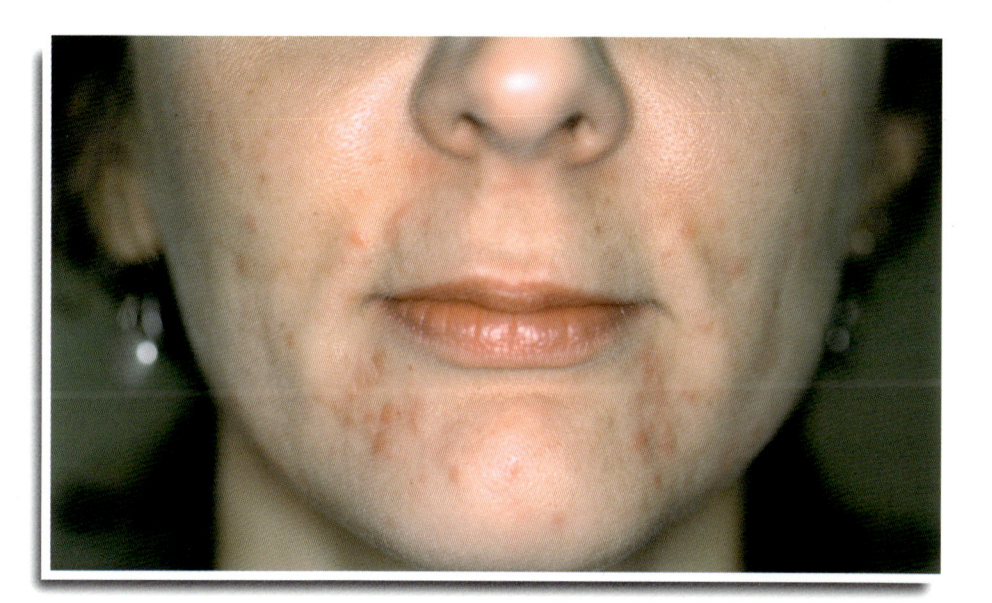

- Typically papular disorder of facial skin associated with topical steroid use
- Can occur in absence of steroid cream use - aetiology unknown
- 1% Hydrocortisone cream or stronger can produce this condition
- Worsening of symptoms with cessation of steroid cream
- Primarily Female 20-30 years old
- Multiple tiny, itchy papules around the mouth
- Can occur around the eyes, spares region immediately adjacent to lips
- Treatment: will respond very slowly with cessation of steroids (months)
- Oral Tetracyclines or topical Metronidazole may be helpful

DERMATITIS - SEBORRHOEIC

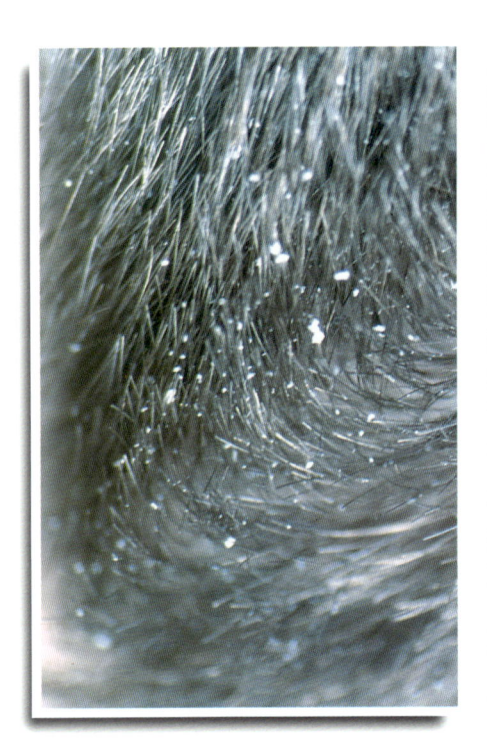

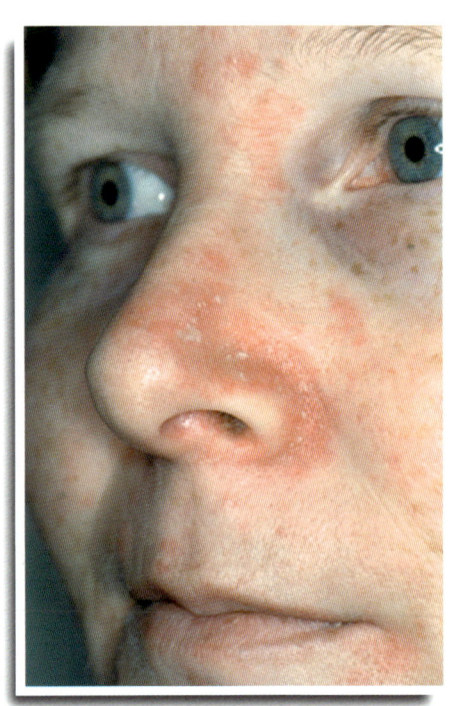

- Common, chronic + distinctive eczema
- Males > Females, 20-50 years, affects 2-5% of population
- Probable infectious agent - Pityrosporum ovale (yeast like micro-organism)
- Dandruff - represents mild condition of scalp
- Red, scaling patches of scalp, eyebrows, forehead, behind ears, front of chest, back + flexures
- Lasts weeks - months - years
- Irritation variable, worsened by sweating, cold climate + stress
- Treatment: anti-fungal shampoo, creams +/- steroid lotion for inflammation
- Coconut or salicylic acid based preparations for thick scales
- Lithium succinate cream may also be helpful

DERMATOFIBROMA
"Histiocytoma"

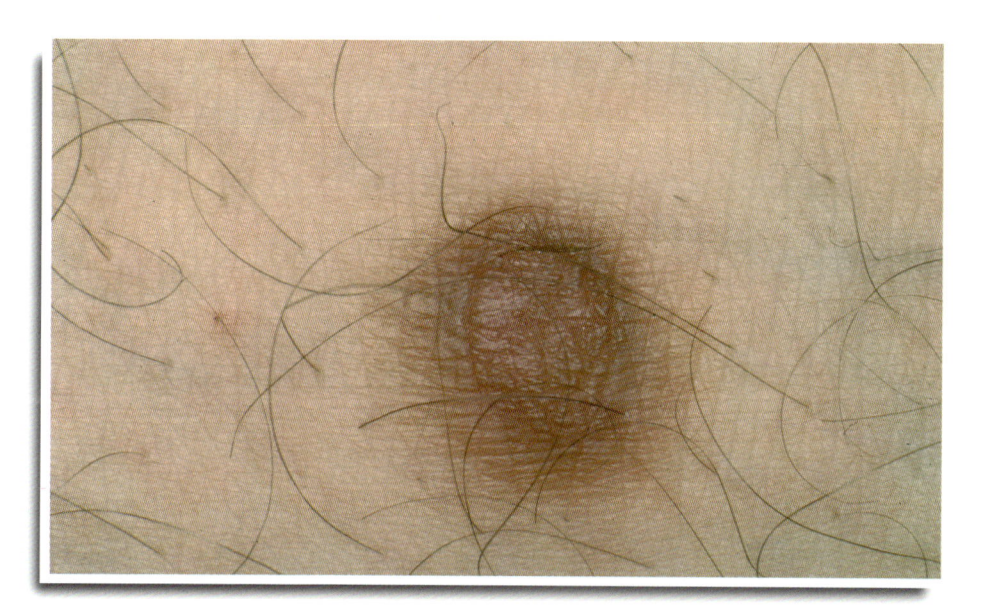

- Benign, firm, fibrous, discrete, dermal nodule
- Female > Male
- Extremities of adults: legs > arms > trunk
- Usually solitary but can be multiple
- Often larger than they appear (iceberg effect)
- Overlying skin lightly pigmented + "dimples" when nodule squeezed (Fitzpatrick's sign)
- Treatment: can be ignored, excise if in doubt, cryotherapy effective + less scarring results

quick reference atlas of dermatology

DERMATOMYOSITIS - JUVENILE

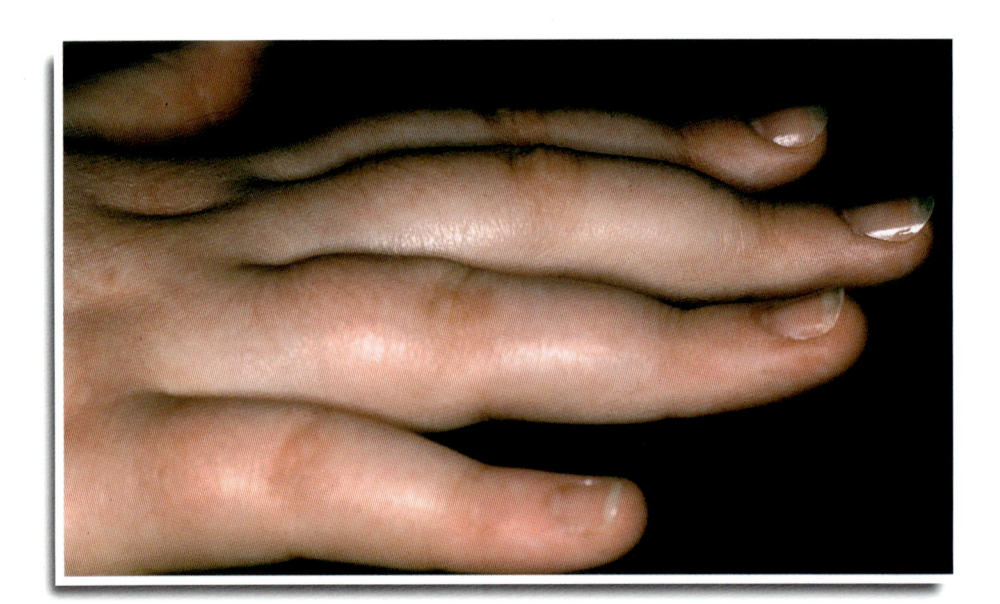

- Inflammatory disorder of skin / striated muscle / possibly GI tract
- Autoimmune, possible viral (Coxsackie B) aetiology. Pathological feature is a vasculitis
- Female > Male (2:1). Peak age approximately 7 years, increased incidence in Spring
- Proximal muscle weakness. Subungual telangiectasia + ragged cuticles
- Skin eruption - violaceous (heliotrope) / oedematous patches → enlarge + coalesce
- Face (primarily periorbital), upper chest, elbows, knees, knuckles (Gottron's papules) + nails
- Calcinosis of tissues can cause ulceration + discharge
- Prognosis variable, spontaneous remission can occur (average 12 months) but can relapse
- Serious complications: florid vasculitis / myocarditis / pulmonary fibrosis
- Diagnosis: ↑CPK / abnormal EMG / muscle biopsy
- Treatment: oral steroids / bed rest in acute phase → physiotherapy
- In adults - 40% have visceral carcinoma (GU, bronchus or breast), carcinoma can develop within 2 years

DERMATOGRAPHISM

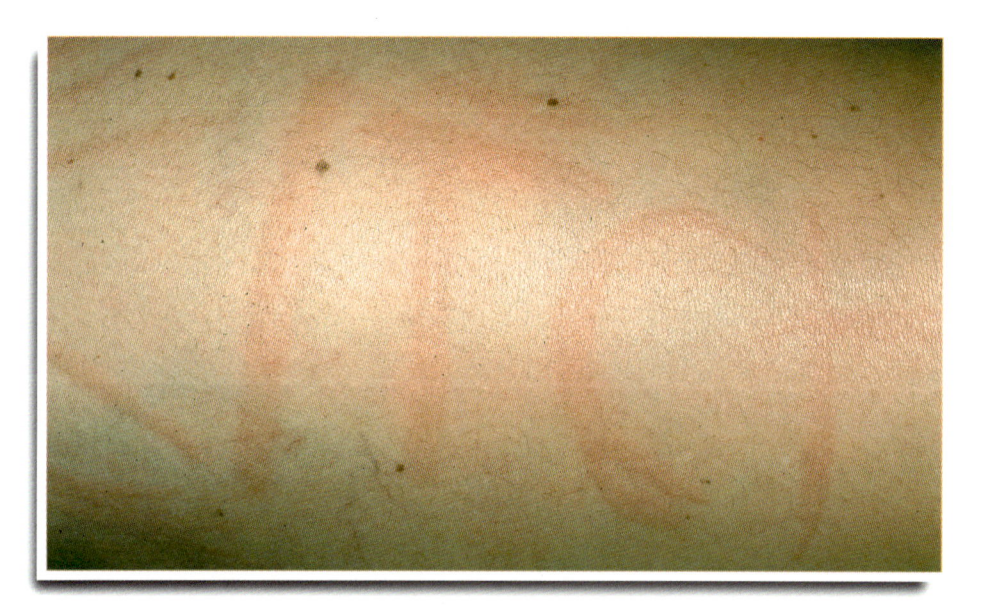

- Physically induced urticaria due to mast cell release of histamine
- Approx. 5% of adults produce exaggerated triple response of Lewis to minor trauma
- Often complain of itching, no associated angio-oedema
- Spontaneous resolution within months → years
- Treatment: if necessary regular long term oral anti-histamines

DRUG REACTIONS

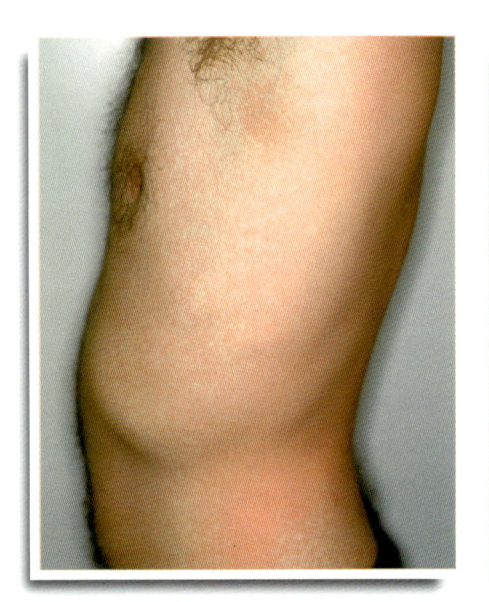

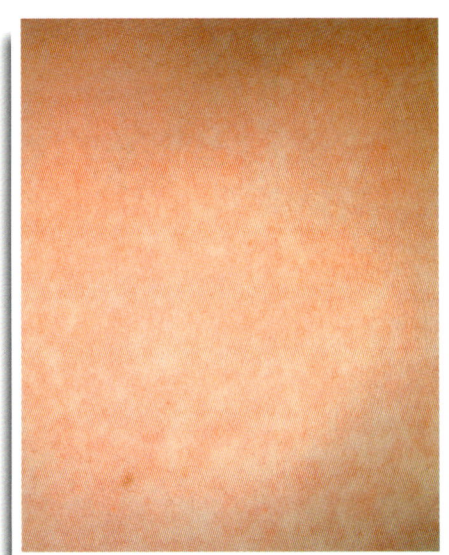

- Adverse, cutaneous reaction to ingested drug e.g. antibiotics, NSAIDs
- Cell mediated immune response
- Morbilliform (measles-like), exanthematous reaction
- Bright red rash, symmetrical, involves trunk, extremities, palms + soles of feet
- Early - within 2-3 days of starting drug in previously sensitised person
- Late - sensitisation occurs during / after completing drug, peak response day 9
- Reaction to penicillin can occur 2 weeks after finishing course
- 10% patients allergic to Penicillin are also sensitive to Cephalosporins
- Treatment: stop drug if reaction severe, oral antihistamines for pruritus, oral steroids if severe

DYSPLASTIC NAEVUS SYNDROME
"Clark Melanocytic Naevus"

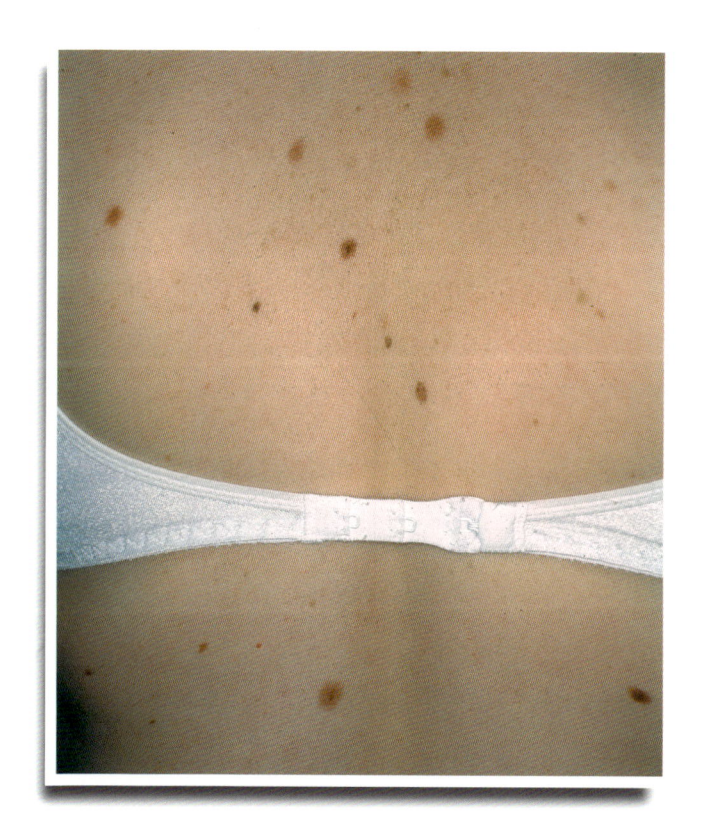

- Familial condition, autosomal dominant, Male = Female, affects 5% white population
- Atypical naevi prone to malignant change (→ malignant melanoma), in teens / early adult life
- Naevi arise prepubertally, new lesions develop + no evidence of regression
- Multiple large, irregular, pigmented naevi, primarily trunk + scalp
- Lesions have irregular edge, vary in size - some > 1 cm
- Contain abnormally large melanocytes + large numbers seen in irregular "nests"
- Abnormal melanocytes activated by sun.
- Higher incidence of malignant change in immuno-suppressed patients with this syndrome
- Treatment: excise → histology, examine all first degree relatives
- 3 - 6 monthly examination with mapping of lesions (photos)
- No sunbathing + sunscreen use when outside
- Patient with 2 relatives with melanoma - 100% chance of malignant change occurring

quick reference atlas of dermatology

ECTHYMA CONTAGIOSUM
"Orf"

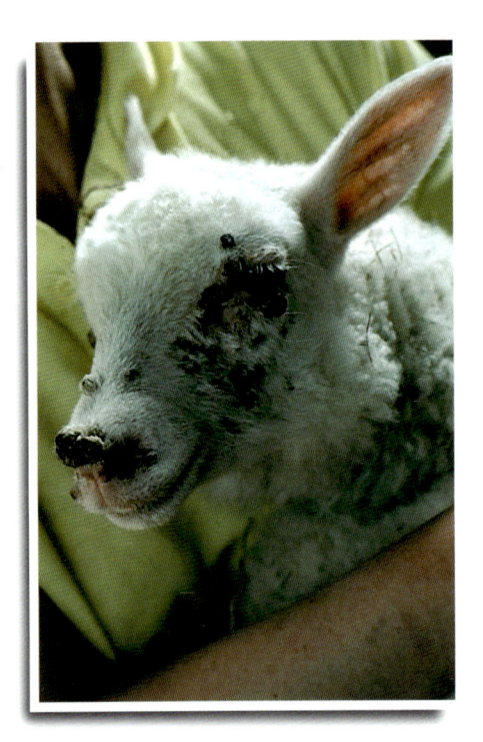

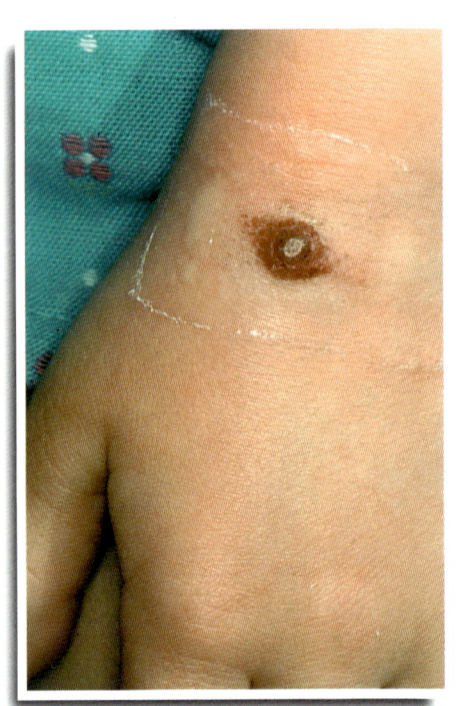

- Contagious, pustular dermatitis, incubation period 5 - 6 days
- Pox virus infection of lambs → sores around mouth + muzzle
- Transmission to human hands via skin abrasions
- Virus can survive on fences / posts for long periods
- Red, purple, off white nodule - looks like a blister but does not contain fluid
- Spontaneous resolution within 4 -5 weeks
- No resultant scarring + patient subsequently immune
- Associated symptoms - lymphadenitis + malaise common, erythema multiforme less common
- Treatment: topical antibiotics can reduce secondary infection

ECZEMA - ATOPIC

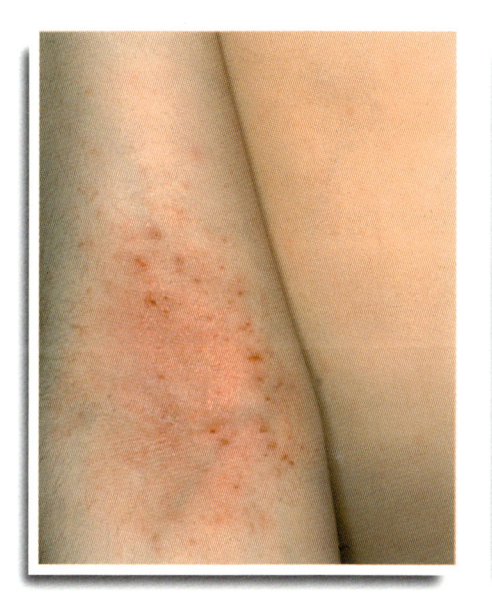

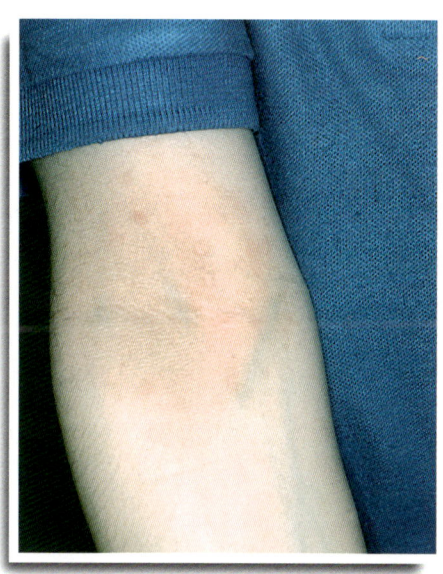

Before therapy

After one week of potent steroid

- Greek : "to boil over"
- Inflammatory disorder of skin responsible for 1/3 of skin disorder consultations
- Remitting / relapsing condition, common in childhood + associated with atopy
- Atopy - group of inherited disorders (asthma, eczema, hayfever + urticaria)
- Onset: eczema 3 - 24 months of age, asthma 3 - 4 years, hayfever + urticaria older children / teens
- Aetiology unknown but inherited tendency (environmental factors important)
- 10% children affected, acute, sub acute + chronic forms
- Psychological / emotional factors aggravate rather than cause
- ↑ IgE in 80% patients, often highly sensitive to house dust mite
- Easily irritated skin, itch is predominant, secondary infection (Staph') common
- Skin tends to be dry (xerosis), ichthyosis + keratosis pilaris in association are common

quick reference atlas of dermatology

ECZEMA - ATOPIC

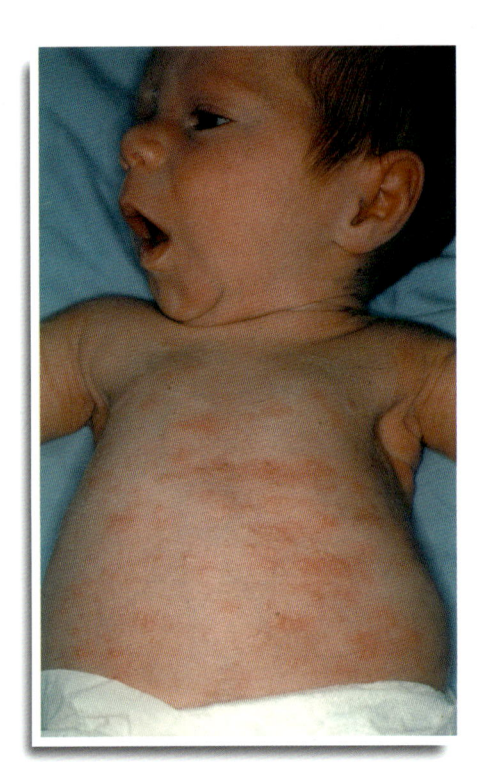

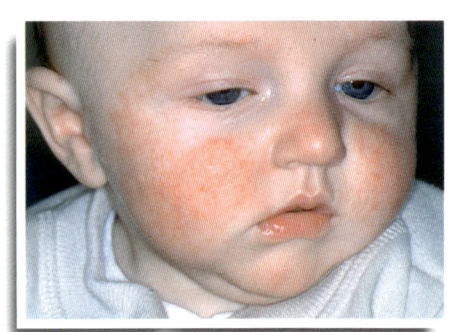

before treatment

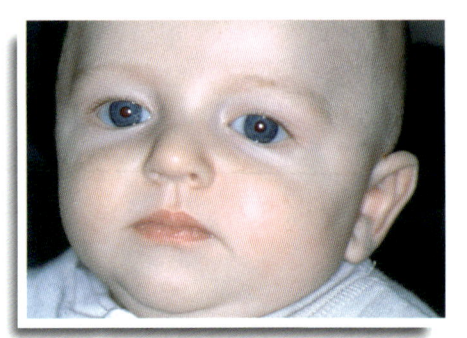

After 3 days of potent steroid

- In infancy - vesicular + weeping, primarily face initially
- In childhood - leathery, dry, excoriated, primarily flexures
- In adults - widespread low grade involvement trunk, face + hands, associated lichenification
- 90% children will outgrow it by teens
- Itch → scratch → inflammation → itch cycle
- Treatment: aim to support rather than cure
- Emollients, topical steroids, occlusion bandages + sedative antihistamines,
- Treat secondary infection, limit house dust mite exposure + self help groups

ECZEMA - DISCOID
"Nummular eczema"

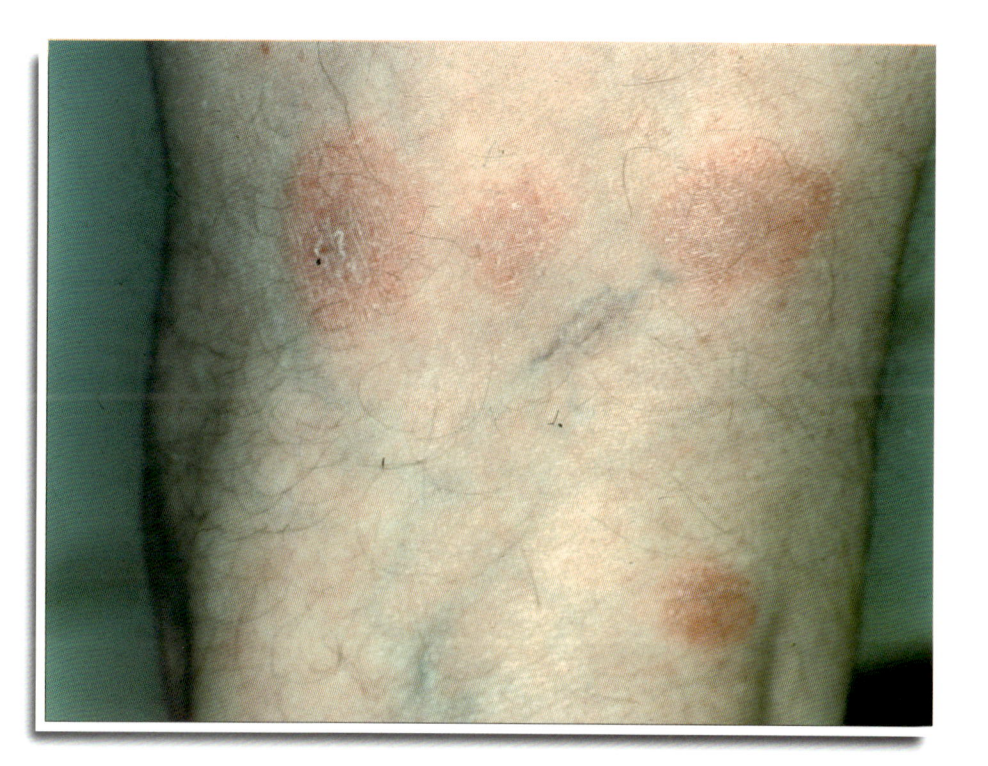

- Latin : "like a coin"
- Endogenous eczema, IgE normal
- No cause evident, stress + Autumn / Winter aggravating factors
- Usually multiple lesions, coin shaped, vesicular or crusted, intensely itchy
- Primarily limbs of middle aged men or hands / fingers of young adults
- Persists for months, Staph' Aureus often cultured from plaques
- Treatment: steroid +/- antibiotics, or tar +/- emollient (increasing tar proportion with time / response)

ECZEMA - VARICOSE
"Stasis Eczema / Gravitational Eczema"

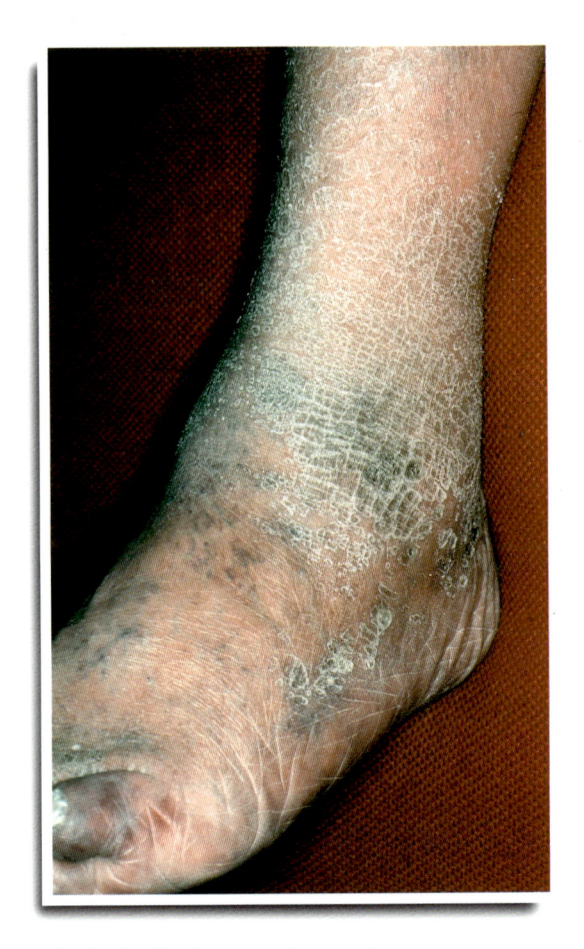

- Confined to lower legs of patients with other signs of venous disease
- Plaques of eczematous skin around ankles + lower legs
- Associated oedema + haemosiderin deposits discolour skin over time
- Treatment: weak topical steroid (ointment) + emollients
- Treatment prevents drying → irritation → scratching → ulceration
- Leg elevation + support bandages / support hosiery
- ↓ weight, ↑ activity / mobility, ↓ oedema
- Encourage walking - improves circulation + reduces venous stasis

EPILOIA
"Tuberose Sclerosis"

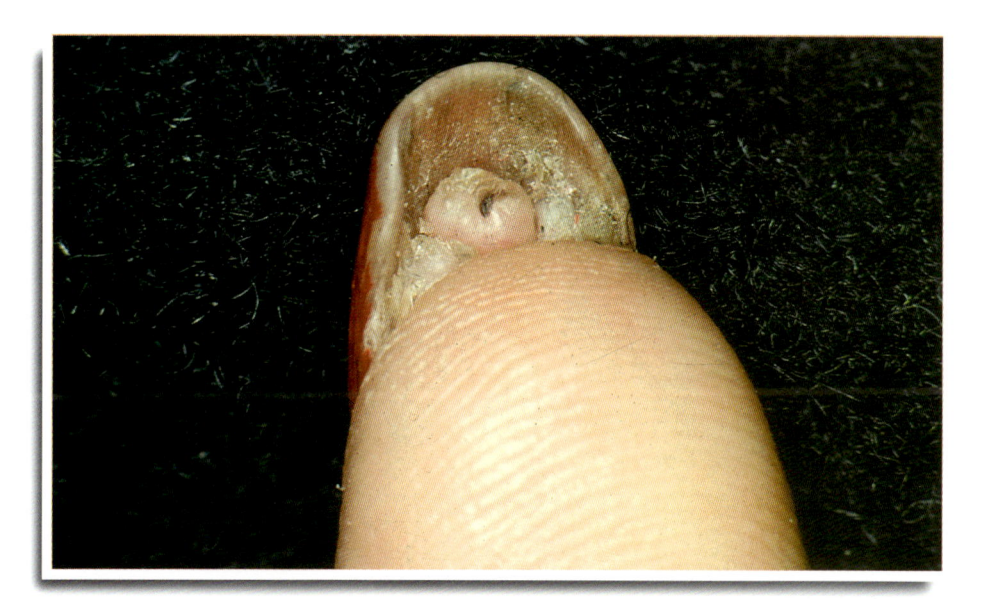

- Serious / uncommon, autosomal dominantly inherited condition
- 50 -70% die before adult hood, skin lesions present in 96% cases
- Reduced fertility, hence transmission through > 2 generations is rare
- Periungual fibromas 22% adults (Koenen's tumours) - pink fleshy lesions at nail folds + subungually
- Adenoma sebaceum: fibrovascular tumour - pink / yellow facial papules, appears 3 -4 years of age
- Ash leaf macules (chagrin patches) - seen with a Wood's lamp, often present at birth
- Cobblestone yellow plaques over base of spine
- Confetti hypopigmentation on legs
- Associated problems - epilepsy, low IQ, hyperplastic gums, renal tumours + gliomas

quick reference atlas of dermatology

ERYSIPELAS

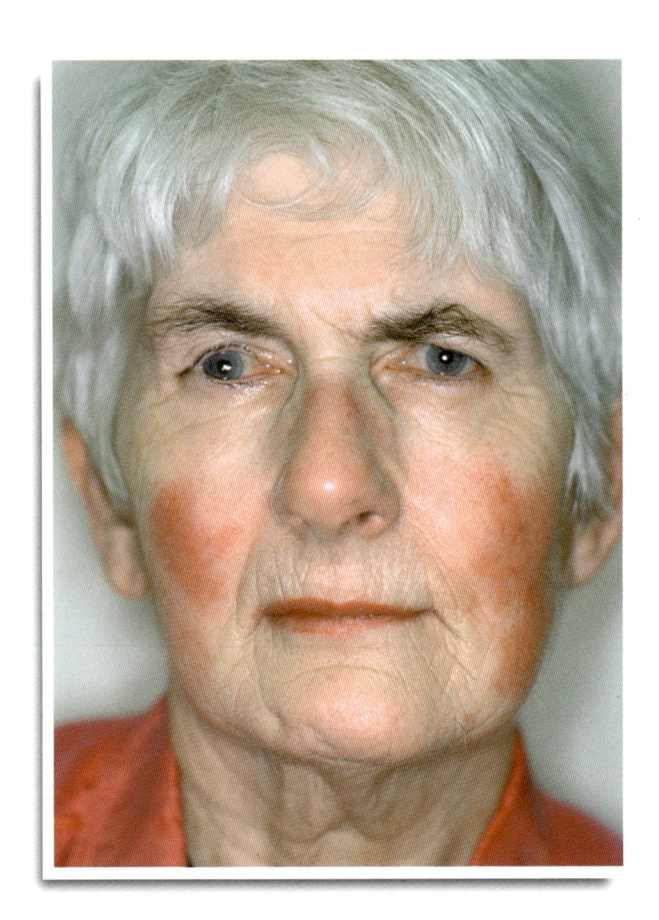

- Group A Beta Haemolytic Strep' infection of upper half of dermis
- Any age, usually in healthy individuals
- Now uncommon but can be life threatening
- Acute onset, rapidly spreading, red, swollen, tender areas with sharply defined edges
- Primarily face or limbs, with or without blistering, no lymphangitis / lymphadenopathy
- Systemic upset include malaise, fever + rigors
- Can have repeated episodes (same area) → persistent lymphoedema
- Treatment: Penicillin urgently, find site of entry if possible (e.g. tinea pedis fissure)
- Support hosiery + low dose antibiotic prophylaxis may reduce recurrences

ERYTHEMA AB IGNE
"Tinker's Tartan"

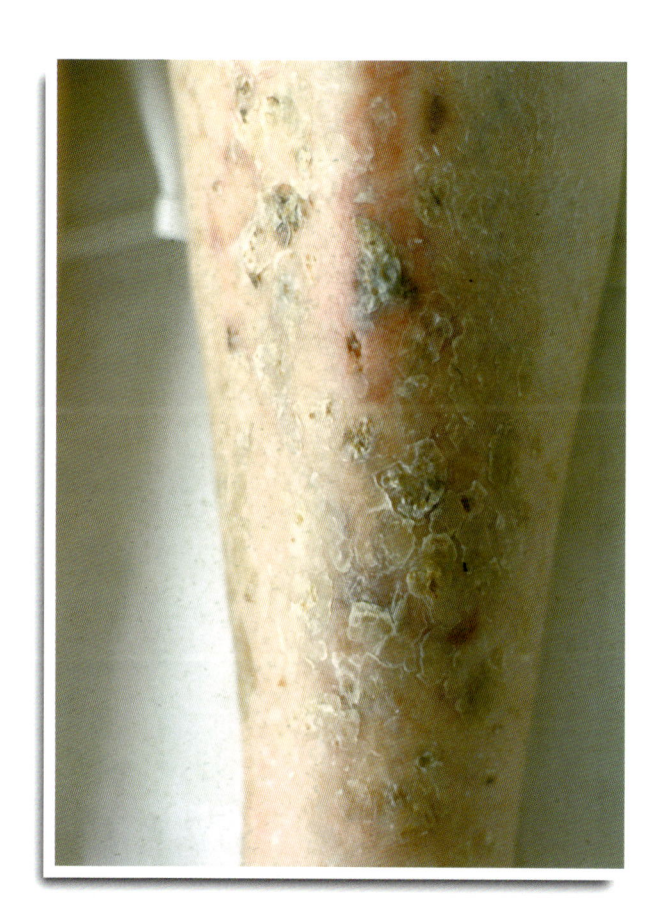

- Reticulate, pigmented erythema with variable scaling
- Primarily lower legs of elderly people, common in northern Europe
- Damage due to long term exposure to local heat source e.g. fire, hot water bottle
- Uncommonly - SCC can arise in area of chronic change

ERYTHEMA INFANTUM
"Fifth Disease"

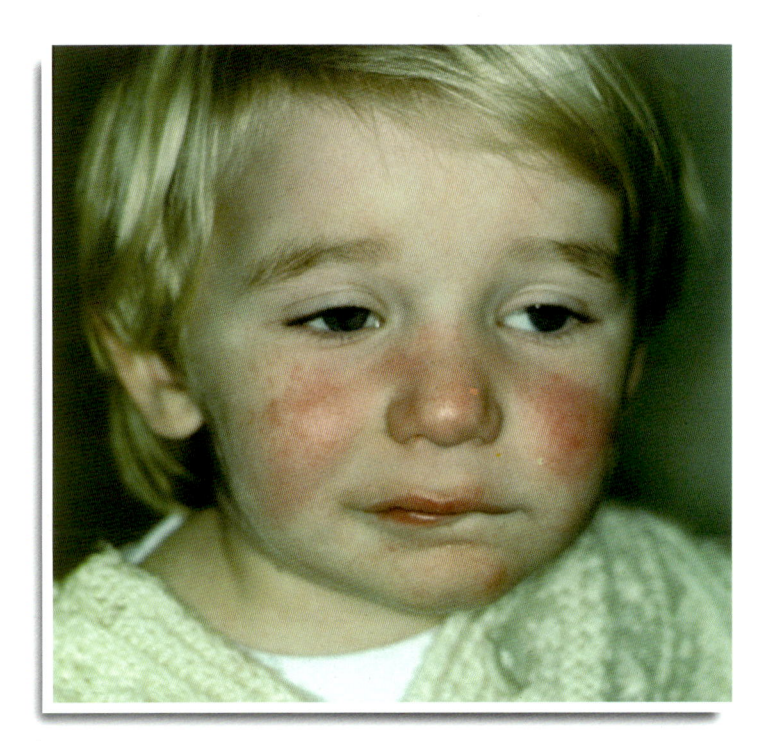

- All ages but primarily childhood exanthema associated with Parvo virus B19
- Droplet / aerosol spread, common late Winter / early Spring
- Oedematous, pink / red, erythematous round / oval plaques on cheeks
- Macules / papules seen elsewhere on body - (lacy + reticulate)
- Incubation period 4 - 14 days, 2 day prodrome of fever, malaise, headache + coryza
- Rash coincides with headache, sore throat, cough, conjunctivitis + nausea
- In adults - systemic effects more pronounced, arthralgia in females (facial rash absent)
- Lasts 5 - 10 days, can recur for weeks or months, triggered by sunlight, exercise, stress + bathing
- Treatment: symptomatic only
- Intrauterine infection with Parvo virus B19 can cause non immune foetal hydrops

ERYTHEMA MULTIFORME

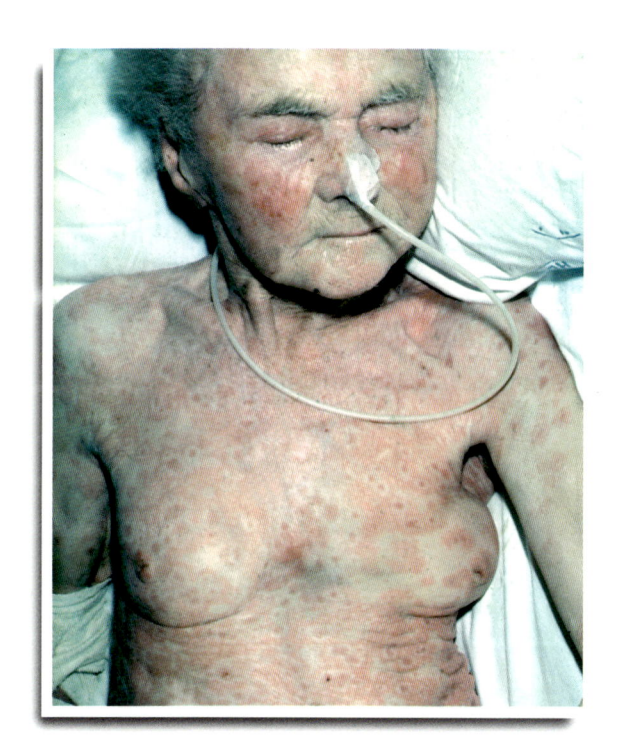

- Reaction to infection (viral / bacterial / fungal), drugs (sulphonamides / NSAIDs / Gold)
- Also seen in pregnancy, malignancy but 50% idiopathic
- Any age, 50% < 20 years, Male > Female, severe bullous form in young boys
- Possibly immune complex mediated, involving epidermis +/- dermis
- Annular, non scaling plaques on palms / soles / forearms / legs, pruritic or painful
- Lesions enlarge, develop rings of different colours with central clearing - typical target lesion
- Appear over 1 - 2 weeks, individual lesions persist for several days
- Can leave short lived hyperpigmentation
- Extreme form - Steven Johnson syndrome with mucous membrane involvement + pyrexia
- Treatment: identify / remove causal factor, antihistamines or short course oral steroids
- Recent findings suggest Cyclosporin may be beneficial
- Recurrent episodes - consider Herpes Simplex - treat with oral antiviral agent

ERYTHEMA NODOSUM

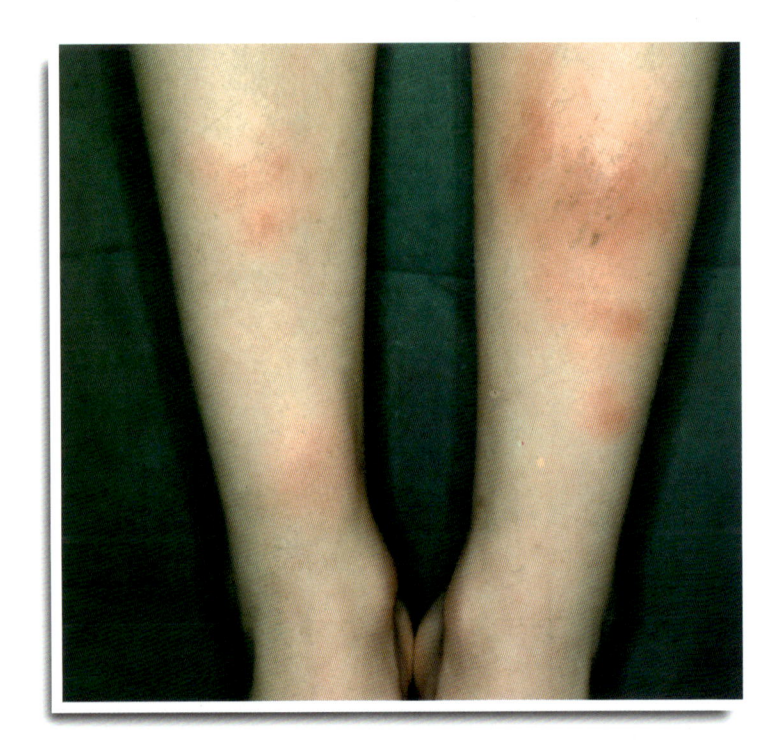

- Painful, red, subcutaneous nodules, 2 - 6 cm diameter on anterior shins, arms thighs + face
- Posterior shin (calf) involvement - consider TB (Erythema Induratum)
- Inflammation of subcutaneous fat, acute reactive panniculitis
- Immunological reaction to various stimuli especially Strep'
- Other associations - anti-TB drugs, Sulphonamides + oral contraceptives,
- Also sarcoidosis, inflammatory bowel disease, 30% unknown,
- Primarily adolescence / adults, Female > Male (3:1), 50% have arthralgia, malaise + fever
- Resolution over 2 - 6 weeks, nodules → bruises → fading. Can recur
- Treatment: treat identifiable cause, analgesia / NSAIDs / pressure bandages to ease leg pain
- Oral steroids if mobility affected

FLEA BITES

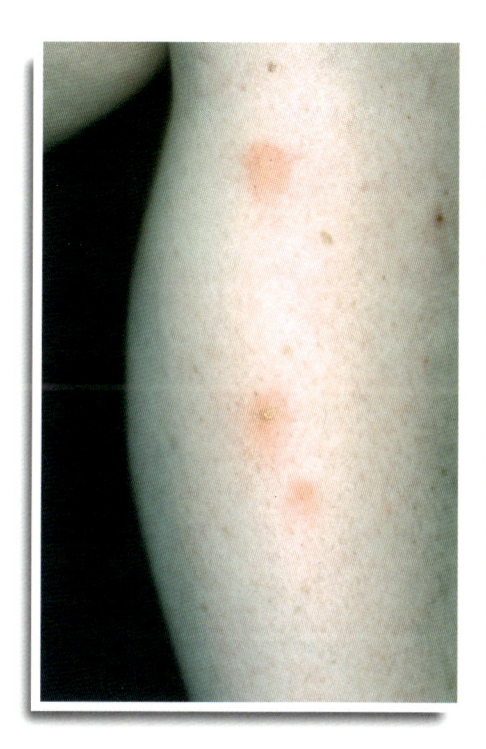

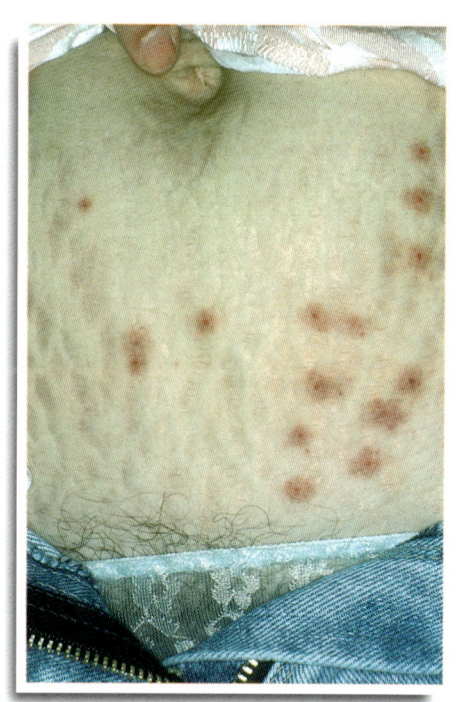

- Skin reaction (immunologically mediated response) to injected arthropodal antigen
- Intensely itchy eruption at site, appears hour - days after bite
- Grouped (usually 3 - "breakfast, lunch + dinner") urticarial papules / vesicles / bullae
- Red, round / domed papules with central punctum
- Primarily legs (ankles → knees), areas where clothing is tight. Perineum + axillae spared
- Persists from days - weeks, more common in children + in Summer
- Heals with hyper / hypo-pigmentation +/- scarring
- Fleas - cat, dog, bird (rarely human), live in carpets / soft furnishings
- Treatment: topical potent steroids or Crotamiton, treat pets + home,

GRANULOMA ANNULARE

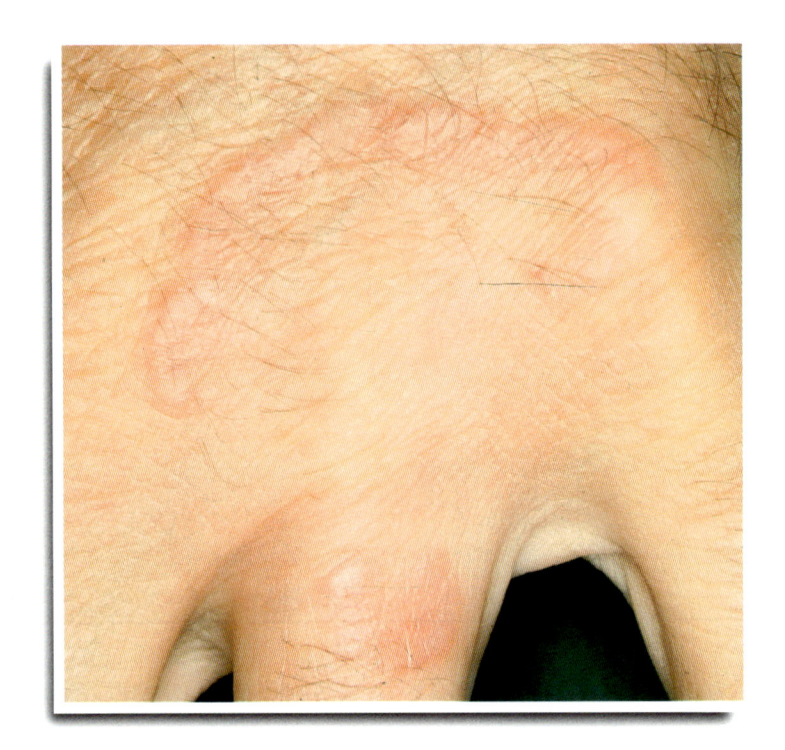

- Local inflammatory process of unknown cause (extensive lesions associated with diabetes)
- Children / young adults, Female > Male (2:1)
- Lesions seen over knuckles, hands + feet
- Dermal nodules fused into a ring shape with beaded border
- Skin coloured / pink on hands, purple elsewhere, no scaling (in contrast to tinea)
- 75% resolve after 2 years, 40% will recur
- Treatment: usually none, intra-lesional Triamcinolone if stubborn
- PUVA for generalised granuloma annulare

GUTTATE PSORIASIS

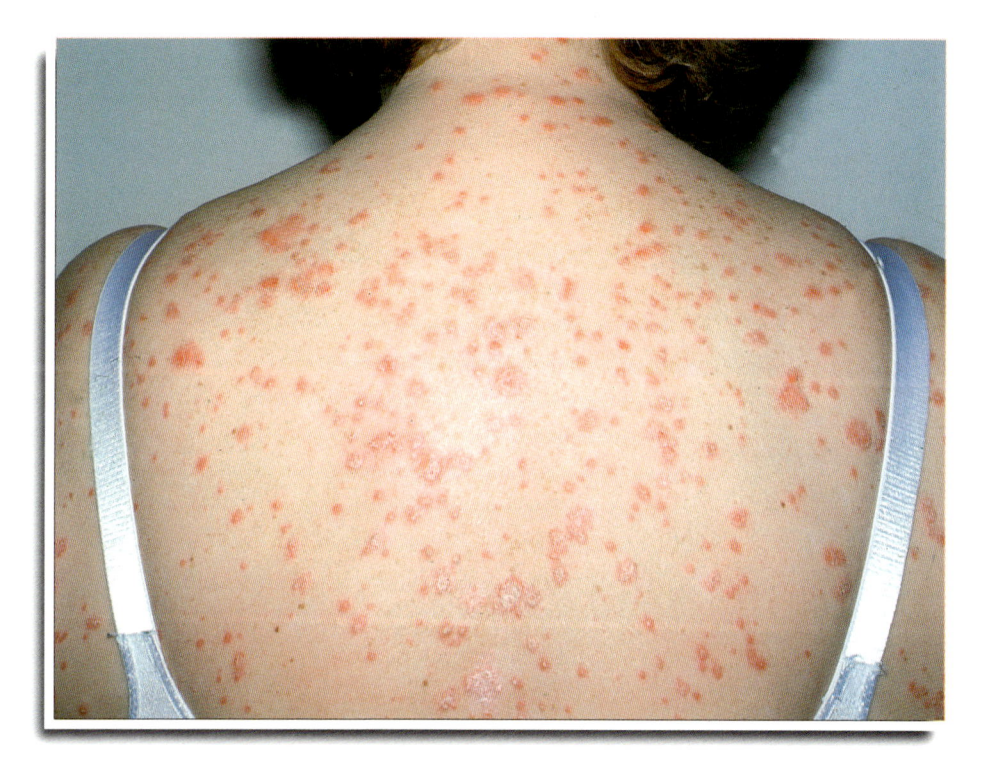

- Latin: "spots that resemble drops". < 2% of all psoriasis seen
- Primarily acute, seen usually in children / young adults
- Bright red, well defined plaques with silver scaling
- 0.5 - 1 cm diameter, all at same stage of development, primarily trunk (spares palms + soles)
- 10 - 14 days after Strep' throat infection, resolves within 2 -3 months, can recur
- May be first manifestation of psoriasis→ becomes chronic (not related to Strep')
- Treatment: antibiotics for throat, emollients + reassurance, do not use Dithranol / tars (→ worse)

HALO NAEVUS
"Sutton's Naevus"

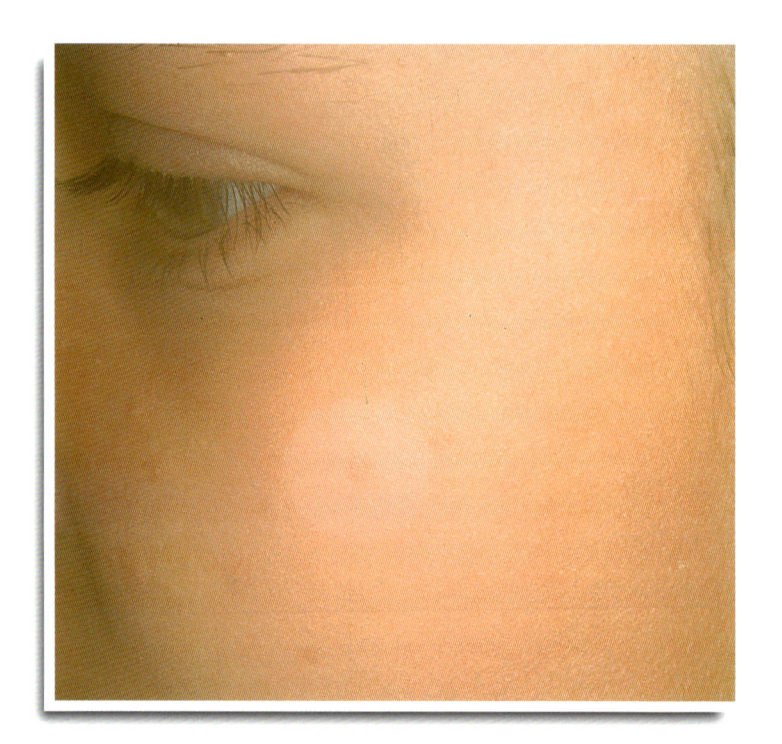

- Appears from birth - 30 years, both sexes + all races
- Autoimmune phenomenon, affected patients have slightly ↑ chance of vitiligo
- A rim of depigmentation appears around one or more benign naevi
- Naevus often involutes months / years later
- Skin eventually repigments over similar time span
- Halo phenomenon can develop around malignant melanoma (always assess naevus!)
- Treatment: reassurance + protect depigmented area from sunburn

HAND, FOOT + MOUTH

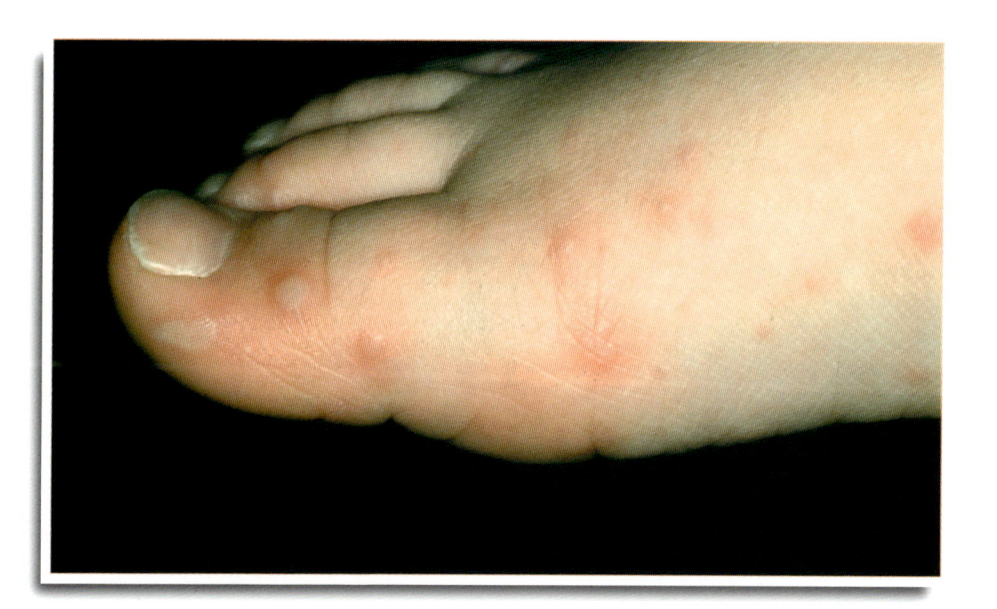

- Highly infectious but mild viral infection due to Coxsackie A16
- Primarily children, also young / middle aged adults, Male = Female
- Droplet spread + faecal contamination
- Epidemics seen every 3 years
- 7 day incubation period, settles within days
- Grey vesicles with red rim on palms, soles + buttocks, oral lesions → often ulcerate (painful)
- Some patients have high fever, malaise, diarrhoea + arthralgia
- Treatment: symptomatic only

HENOCH SCHONLEIN PURPURA
"Anaphylactic Purpura"

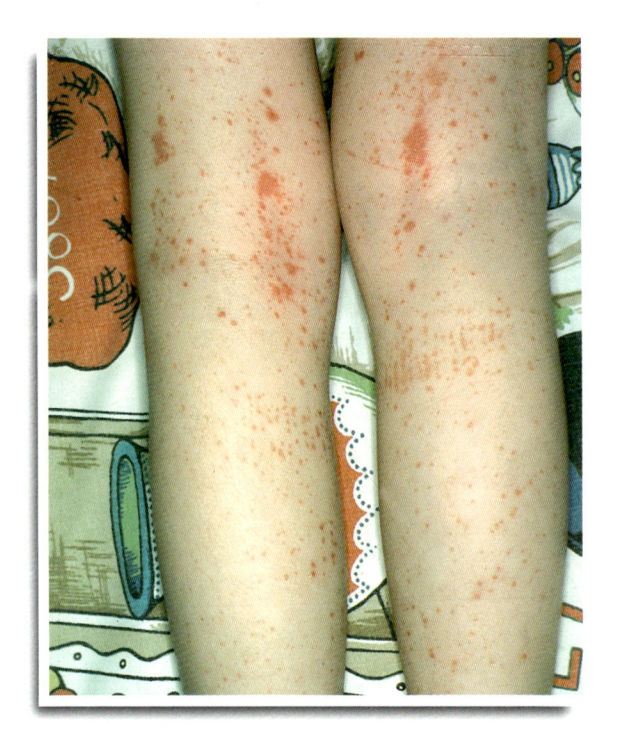

- Immune complex mediated hypersensitivity vasculitis due to Group A Strep' + viruses
- Idiopathic in 50%, primarily children < 7 years but can occur at any age, Male > Female
- Palpable haemorrhagic skin lesions with raised purpuric centre
- Numerous, primarily buttocks + legs, can → trunk + arms
- Associated symptoms - fever, arthritis of ankles / knees, facial oedema + swelling dorsum hands
- Renal involvement → microscopic haematuria
- Serious complications - glomerulonephritis → nephrotic syndrome → renal failure (rare)
- Also abdo' pain (70%) → bowel ischaemia (rare) with bloody diarrhoea
- Treatment: identify + treat Strep' if cause, assess urine for blood + protein (monitor renal function)
- No treatment for skin lesions as resolve in 1 - 3 weeks

HERPES SIMPLEX LABIALIS
"Cold Sores"

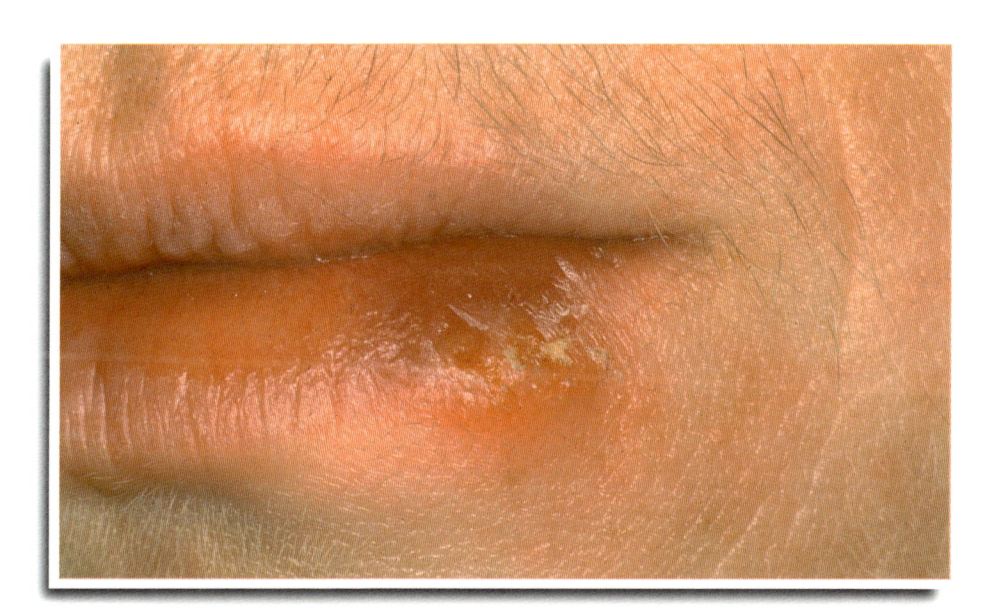

- Latin: Herpes = "to creep" Herpes Simplex hominis type I (majority).
- Spread by direct inoculation
- Initial infection - age 1 - 4 years (by 9 years > 10% have infection)
- Symptoms - fever, vesicles on lips, mouth ulceration, sore throat + lymphadenopathy
- Spontaneous resolution 1 - 2 weeks
- Secondary eruption - older children, recurrent into adult life, less frequent with time
- Always milder than primary infection, eruptions preceded by prodromal discomfort + paraesthesia
- Grouped vesicles on red erythematous background → burst → dry → crust within 10 days
- Lesions usually on face erupting in same area each time. No scarring
- Virus latent in sensory ganglia, precipitants - sun, cold, menstruation + fever
- Treatment: often none or antiviral cream

HERPETIC WHITLOW

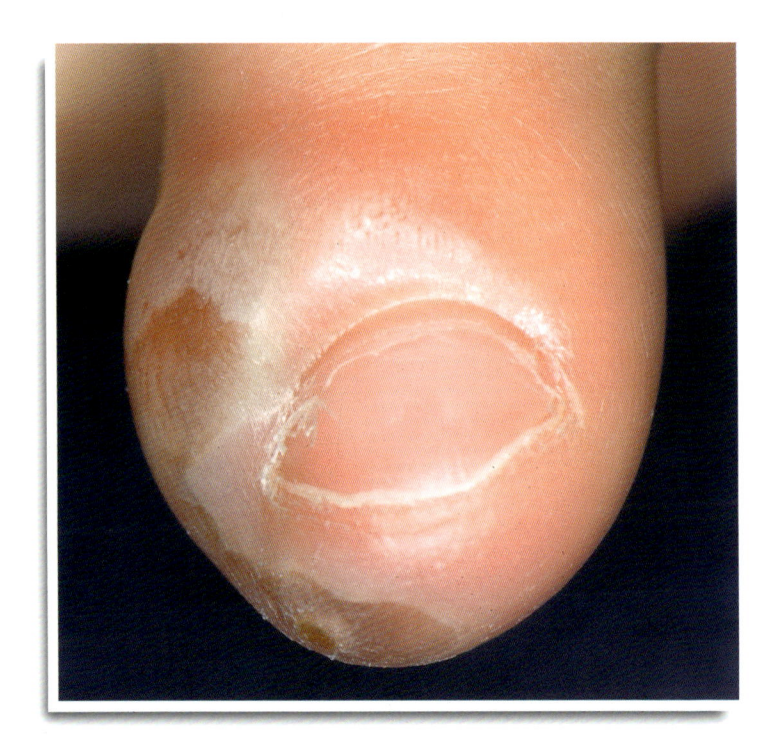

- Whitlow : any pussy inflamation of end of digit
- Example of direct inoculation with H. Simplex virus
- Painful, pus filled blisters on erythematous / oedematous base
- Usually tip of finger, often in medics nursing patients with H. Simplex
- 2 weeks to resolution, recurrence common
- Treatment: primary attack - consider systemic antiviral, cream for recurrences

quick reference atlas of dermatology

HERPES ZOSTER
"Shingles"

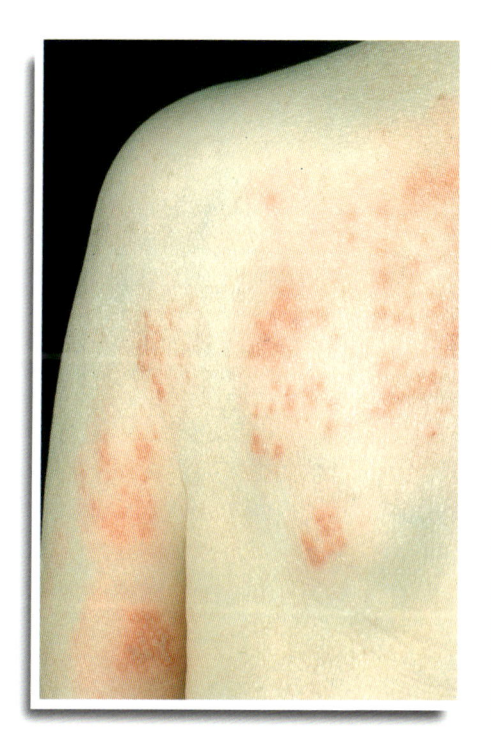

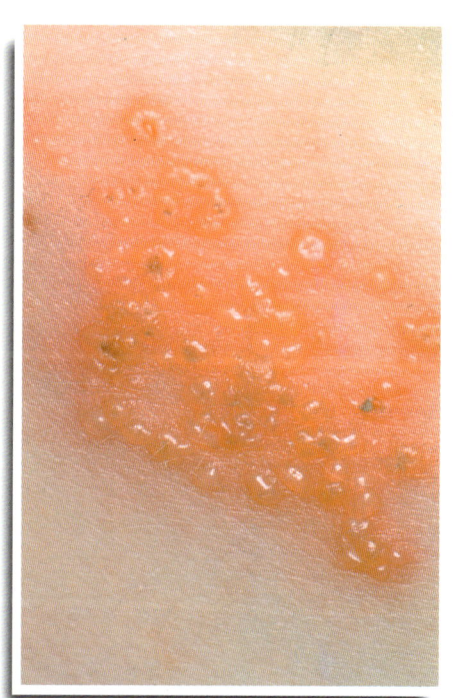

- Vesicular eruption in 1+ adjacent, unilateral dermatomes. 60% > 50 years, 5% < 15 years old
- Reactivation of Varicella virus (chicken pox) - dormant in dorsal root ganglion
- Primarily thoracic or ophthalmic division of trigeminal nerve
- Initially - pain / hyperaesthesia in dermatome, 1 - 14 days before appearance of vesicles
- Red papules → vesicles → pustules → crusting → healing in 3 - 4 weeks
- Can leave depressed / pigmented scarring
- Complications: disseminated infection with haemorrhagic + necrotic lesions if immuno-compromised
- Others: secondary infection, motor nerve involvement → paralysis (rare)
- Post herpetic neuralgia (elderly) can last months / years → depression
- Treatment: often none, analgesia +/- oral antiviral if started within 72 hours
- N.B. vesicles on tip / side of nose = corneal involvement → ophthalmological referral

quick reference atlas of dermatology

ICHTHYOSIS VULGARIS

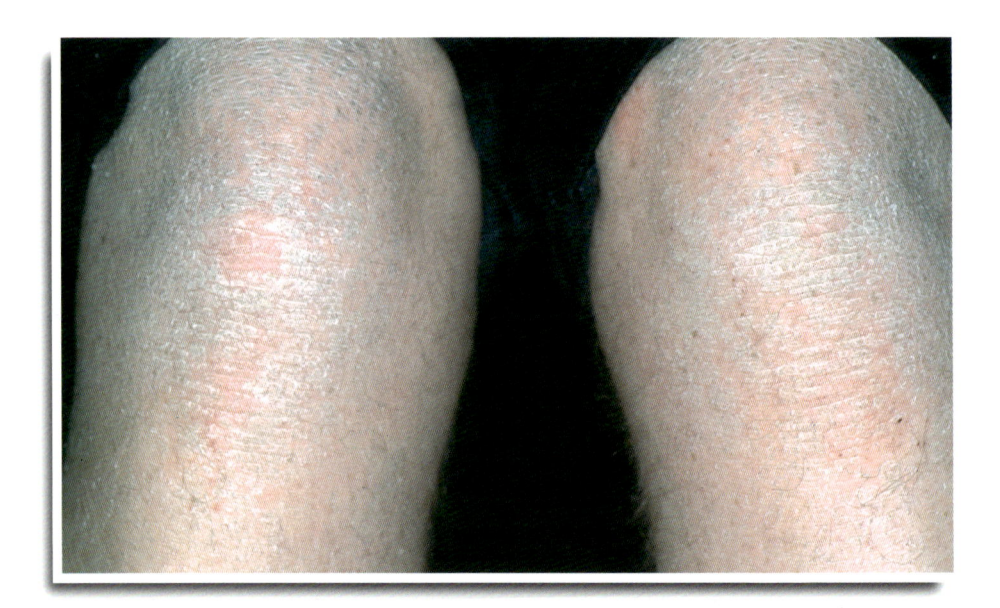

- Greek : Ichthyosis = "a fish"
- Ichthyoses - group of disorders → marked scaling without inflammation
- Ichthyosis vulgaris - 1:300 people affected, autosomal dominant inheritance
- Mild dryness, large, grey / light brown shield like scales, few symptoms
- Mostly on limbs, can be seen on major flexures + face
- Increased palm creases, Keratosis Pilaris commonly seen on limbs
- Hair, teeth + nails normal
- Develops in first years of life, lessens in adulthood but never fully resolves
- Appears to be helped by warm weather, possibly worse if associated with atopic eczema
- Treatment: palliative emollients + urea / lactic acid containing preparations helpful

IMPETIGO

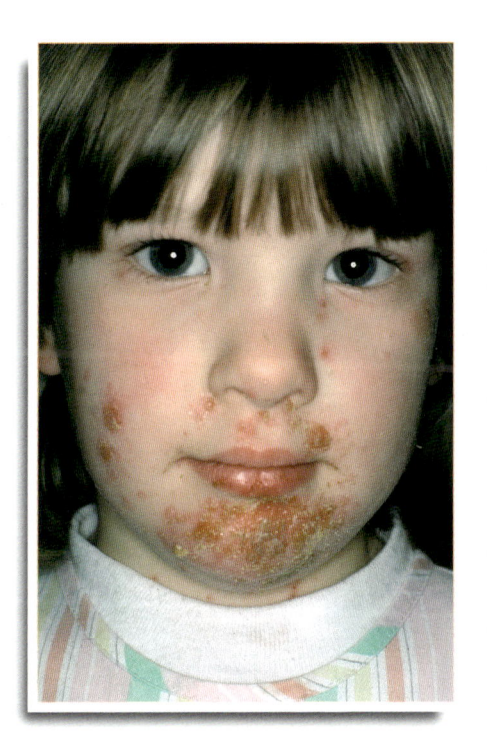

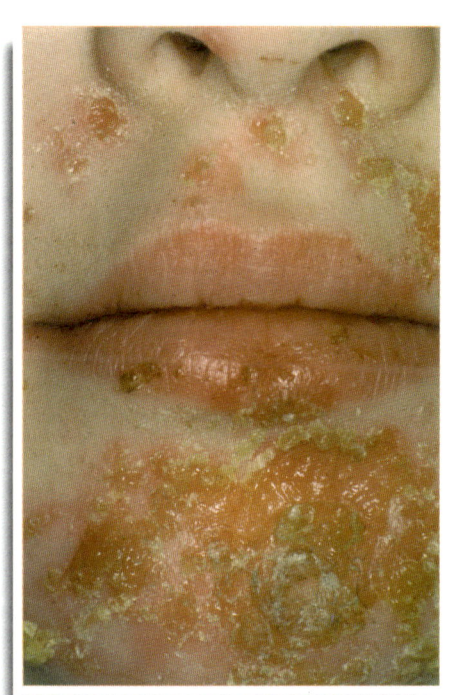

- Common, superficial, highly contagious Staph' or Strep' infection of skin
- If penetrating dermis with ulceration + thick crusting then known as ecthyma (associated with Strep')
- Vesicles → annular erosions 1 - 2 cm diameter, with erythematous base and gold crust (aureus = gold)
- Occurs anywhere on body, primarily face. Impetigo of scalp associated with headlice
- Lesions often multiple, infection enters via skin trauma
- Resolves within 1 week if treated promptly
- Complications - glomerulonephritis (rare) due to Strep', Impetiginised eczema / H. Simplex / Scabies
- Treatment: remove crusts with arachis oil / olive oil / sunflower oil
- Minor limited lesions - treat promptly with topical antibiotics or systemic antibiotics if extensive
- If recurrent - possible Staph' carrier within family (20 - 40 % adults nasal carriers) → identify + treat

INSECT BITES

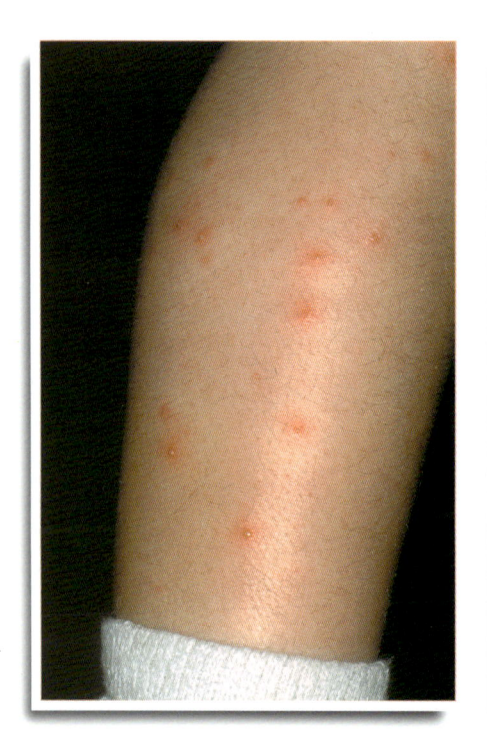

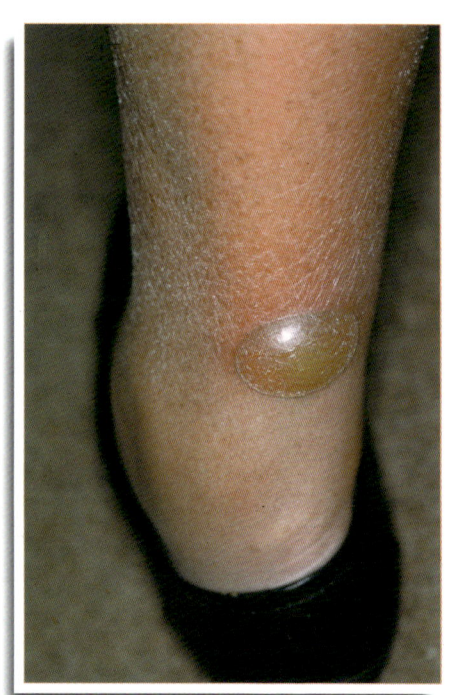

- Itchy papules with central punctum, blistering less commonly occurs
- Skin changes due to pharmacologically injected substance + sensitisation reaction to antigen
- Common site - lower legs, mosquito + midge bites - insects suck blood for food
- Mosquitoes feed from evening to day break, midges feed all day
- Mosquitoes attracted by carbon dioxide in breath + other chemicals in body odour
- Treatment: Calamine lotion, oral antihistamines + prophylactic insect repellent

JUVENILE PLANTAR DERMATOSIS
"Toxic Sock Syndrome"

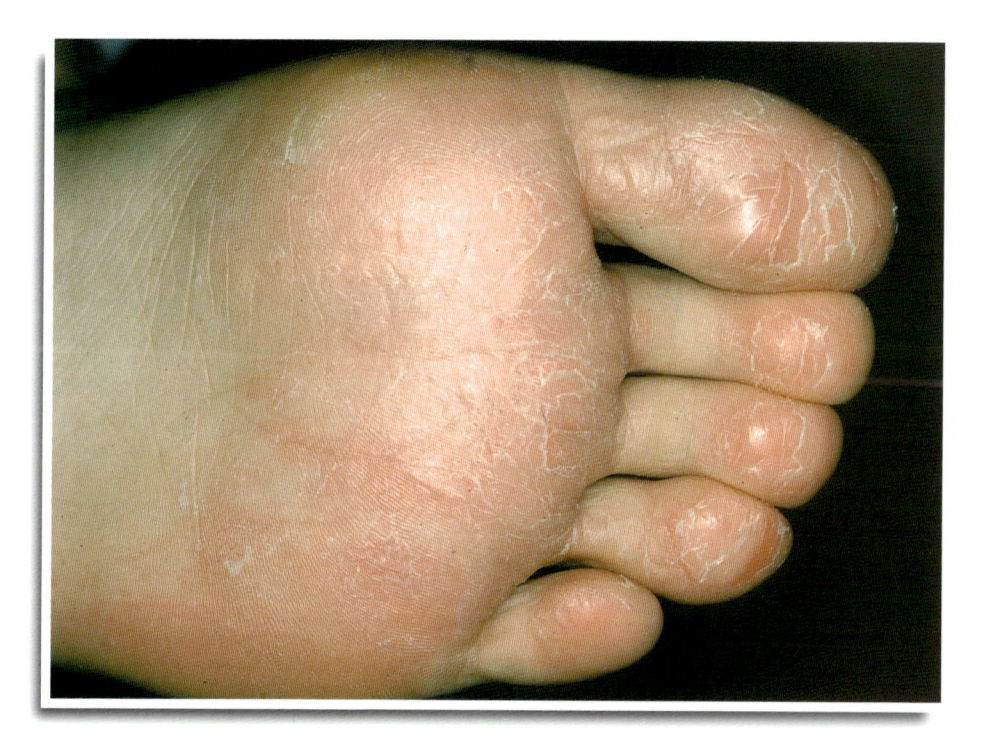

- Dry erythema with fissuring, unique to children + teenagers (8 - 14 years)
- Confined to plantar forefoot + heel (to lesser degree)
- Painful condition, glazed red appearance → cracking → peels + bleeds, toe spaces typically spared
- Only described in last 30 years. ?due to modern shoes e.g. trainers + hosiery
- Link with atopy controversial, role of friction + sweating unclear
- Treatment: charcoal / cork insoles, cotton / wool socks to absorb sweat
- Avoid long term wearing of occlusive footwear especially if synthetic material or lining
- Emollient +/- lactic acid, or urea based - as good as topical steroids

KAPOSI'S VARICELLIFORM ERUPTION
"Eczema Herpeticum"

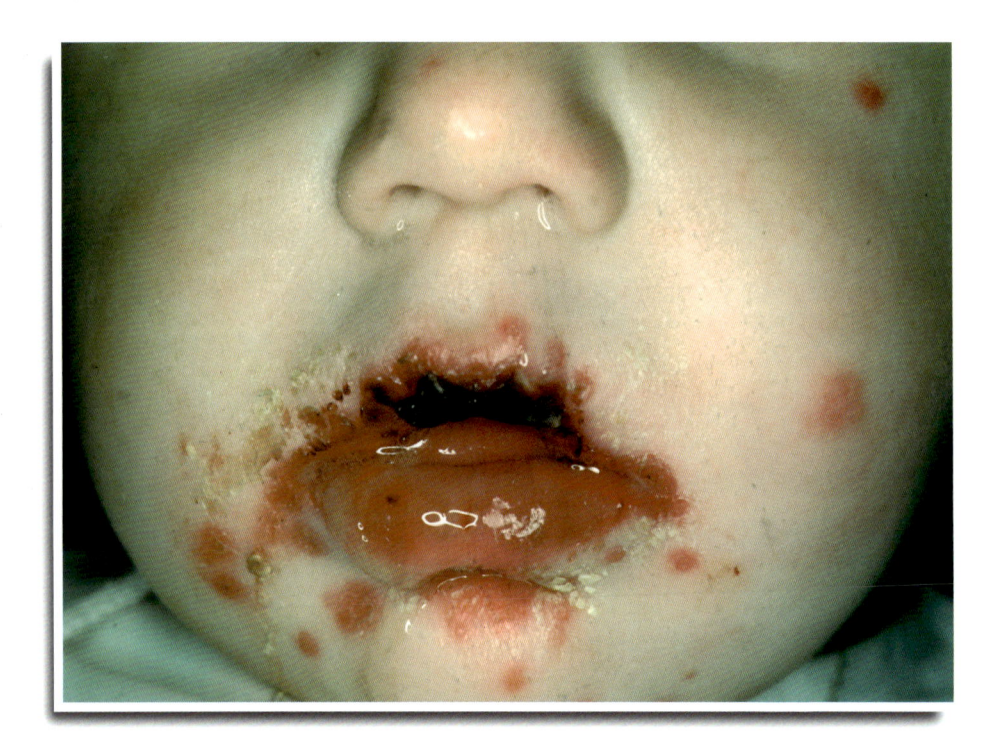

- Widespread cutaneous Herpes Simplex virus infection in underlying skin condition e.g. eczema
- Children > adults, involves face / neck / trunk, also seen with Vaccinia + Coxsackie virus
- Can be primary (with fever + lymphadenopathy) or recurrent
- Primary infection often from parental H. Simplex labialis (resolves within 2-3 weeks)
- Recurrent attacks often less severe + short lived
- Lesions begin in abnormal skin + extend peripherally for weeks to involve normal skin
- Umbilicated vesicles → punched out erosions → confluent erosions → large raw areas
- Itchy skin becomes painful + tender
- Systemic spread in immuno-compromised patient is associated with 10 - 50% mortality
- Treatment: mild cases none needed, oral antiviral for 7 days (i.v. if severe)
- Oral antibiotics for Staph' impetiginisation

KELOID

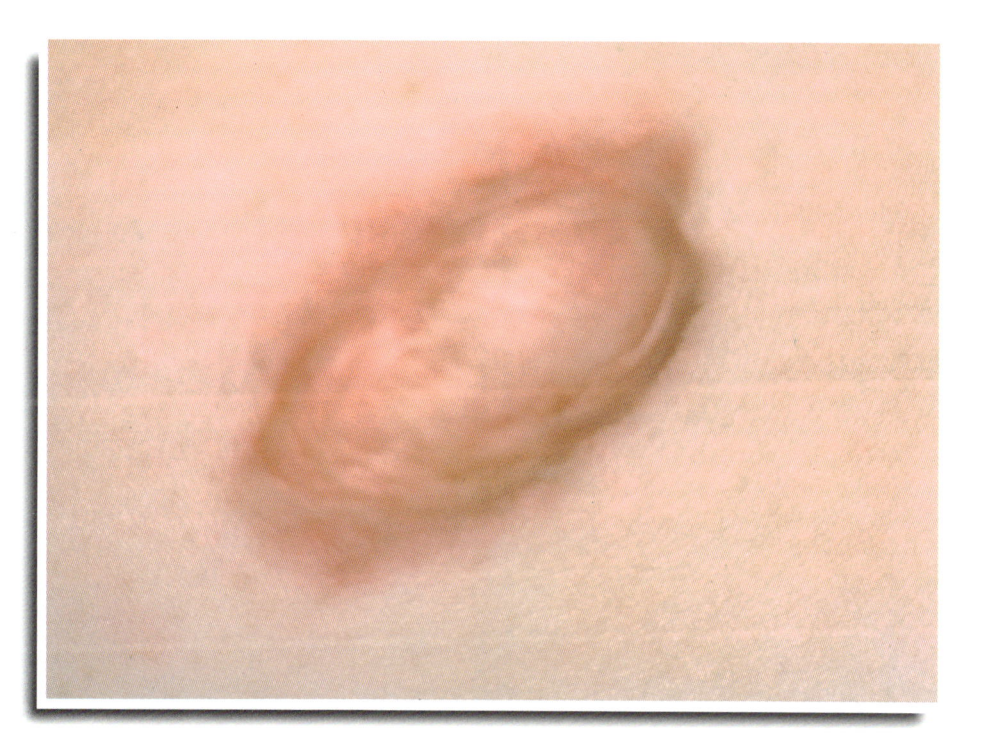

- Hypertrophic scar = overgrowth of scar tissue confined to site of injury, regresses in time
- Keloid scar = overgrowth of dense fibrous tissue beyond injury site, often with claw like extensions
- Primarily 3rd decade, Male = Female, may be familial, common in Negroes
- Common sites: shoulders, front of chest (can occur spontaneously here) + earlobes
- Papules → nodules → large tuberous lesions
- Encouraged by infection / foreign material / wounds or incisions made across creases
- Often irritant, can be painful, frequently cosmetically ugly. Cryotherapy can reduce bulk
- Treatment: patients prone to keloid - avoid cosmetic procedures e.g. body piercing
- Triamcinolone injection to existing lesion or into site of elective surgery of keloid former
- Avoid excision, if impossible - irradiate with Iridium immediately post op

KERATOACANTHOMA

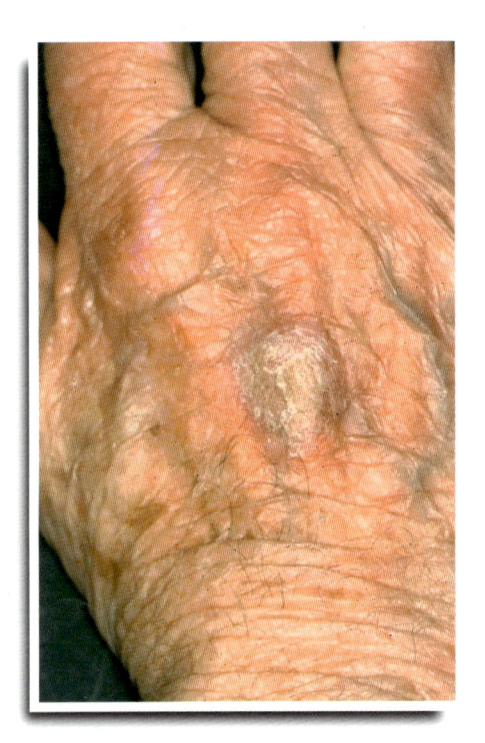

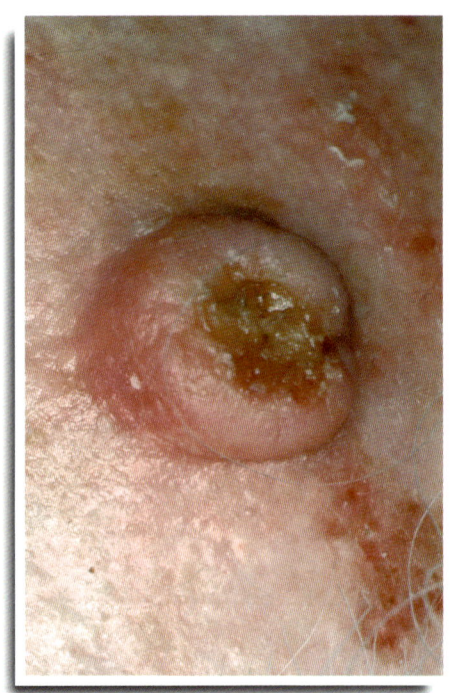

- Rapidly growing, benign tumour of sun exposed area, usually singular, rarely multiple
- Also seen due to mineral oil exposure, therapeutic immuno-suppression, skin treated with UV + tar
- Primarily Caucasians > 50 years, rare < 20 years, Male : Female (2:1)
- 70% appear on face, most of rest on upper limbs
- Symmetrical with erythematous circumference + horny volcano like centre
- Looks like BCC but rapid growth and keratin plug distinguishes it
- Grows for 3 months → static → spontaneous regression → some scarring
- Small number can → SCC
- Treatment: formal excision to distinguish from SCC
- Curettage + cautery (before natural regression begins) if lesion too large to easily excise,
- Any recurrence → re-curette / radiotherapy / formally excise

KERATOSIS PILARIS

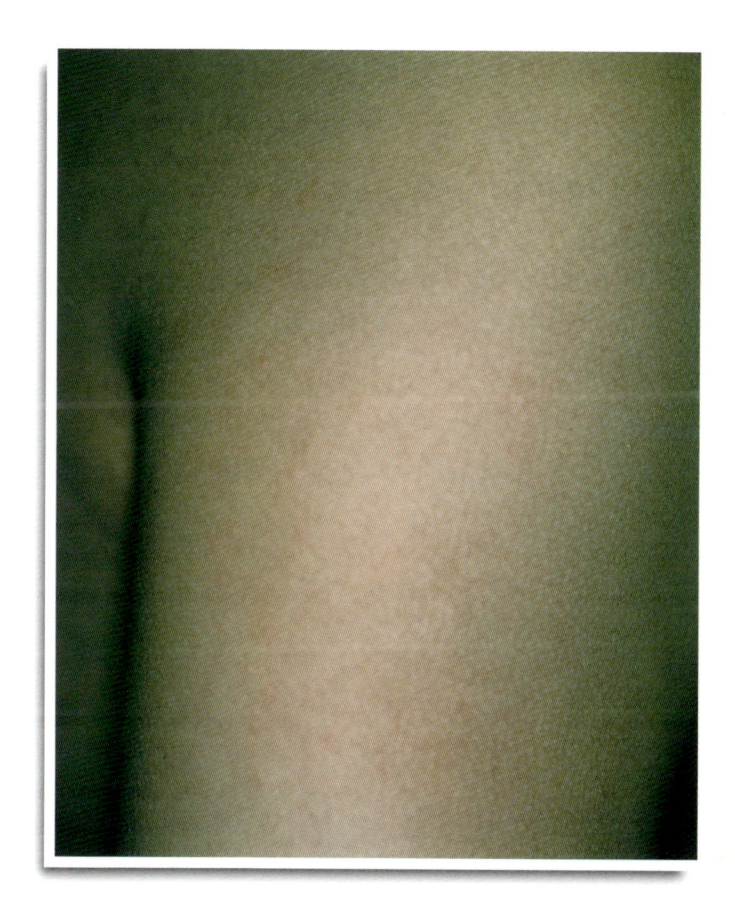

- Perifollicular hyperkeratosis - associated with Ichthyosis Vulgaris + atopy
- Cause unknown, autosomal dominant inheritance
- Common in childhood / adolescence
- Small skin coloured / pink horny spines, symmetrical, primarily shoulders, upper arms + thighs
- Hair follicles blocked by horny plugs, skin feels rough like sandpaper
- Keratosis pilaris in childhood can affect cheeks
- Improves with age, can leave pitted scars + hair loss from eyebrows
- Improves in Summer, humid climates + with increasing age
- Treatment: as for ichthyosis vulgaris - emollients + keratolytics helpful but not curative

LICHEN PLANUS

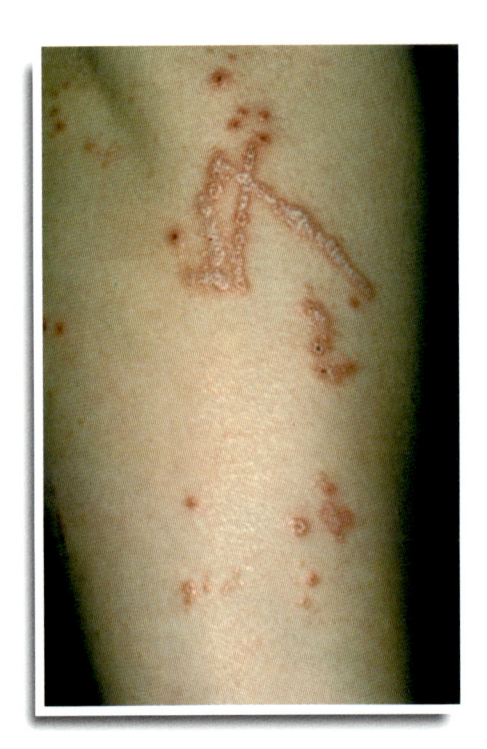

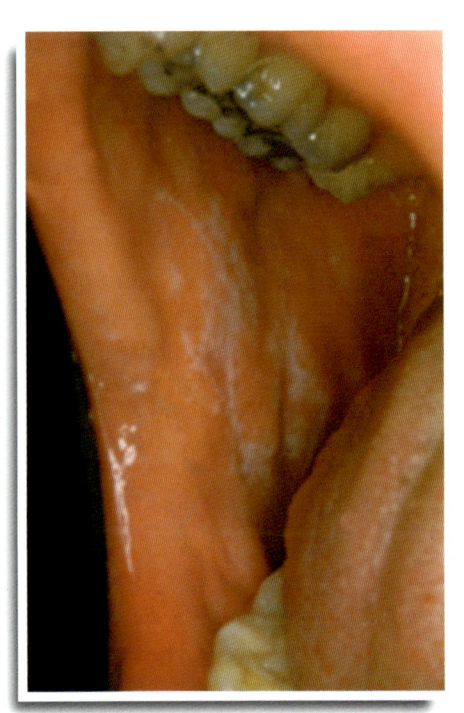

- Latin: planus = flat. Very itchy papular rash occasionally ‡ scaling plaques
- Inflammatory dermatosis cause unknown, Female > Male, age 30 - 60 years
- Primarily extremities, flexor aspect wrists + trunk
- Seen along lines of trauma / scars - Koebner phenomenon (also seen with psoriasis + planar warts)
- Papules - small, polygonal, flat topped, mauve / violaceous
- White lines on lesions are called Wickham's striae
- White asymptomatic streaking seen on buccal mucosa in 50% patients, can ulcerate + last years
- Skin lesions last months, (overall, approximately 18 months) → hyperpigmentation after resolution
- Nails usually normal but may have longitudinal groves → nail bed destruction
- Some drugs cause LP like eruption - gold, antimalarials, thiazides, B blockers, ACEs + Penicillamine
- Treatment: stop causative drug, potent topical steroids relieve itching + flatten plaques
- PUVA can reduce itching + clear lesions. 1:6 patients have a recurrence

LICHEN SIMPLEX CHRONICUS

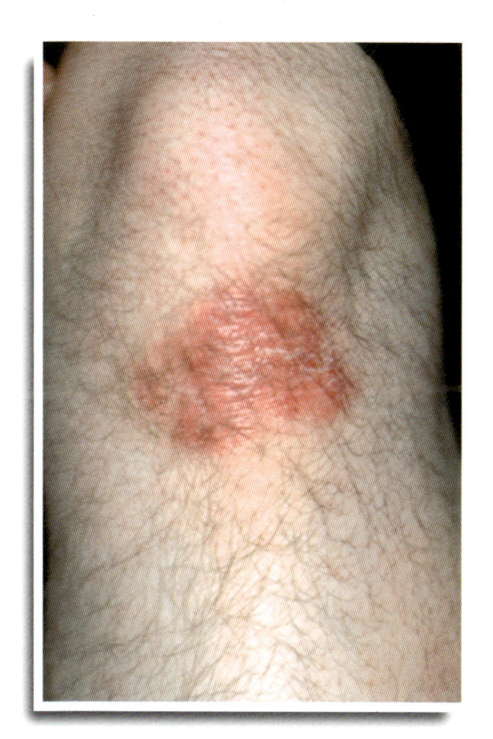

- Localised neurodermatitis seen in Female >> Male, > 20 years of age
- Usually single, fixed, lichenified plaque with exaggerated skin markings
- Involves neck (female), legs (male) + perineum in both sexes
- Skin damaged by repeated scratching / rubbing due to habit / stress
- Rubbing becomes automatic + unconscious
- Treatment: explanation, potent steroids + occlusion to prevent scratching
- If severe / resistant consider intra-lesional Triamcinolone (beware atrophy)

quick reference atlas of dermatology

MEASLES

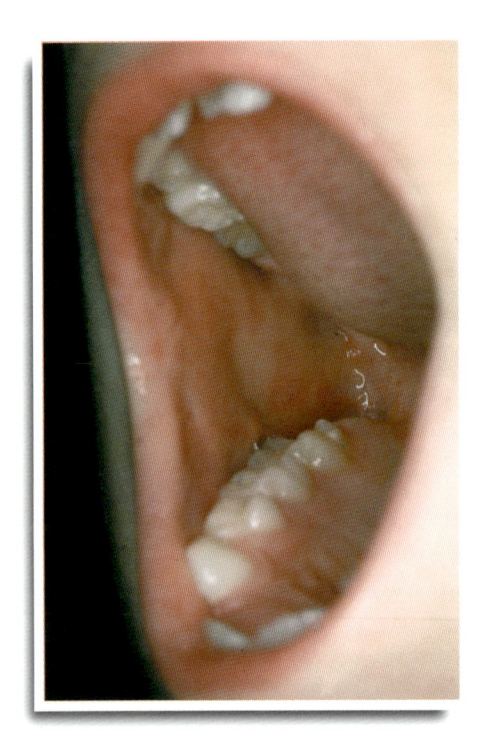

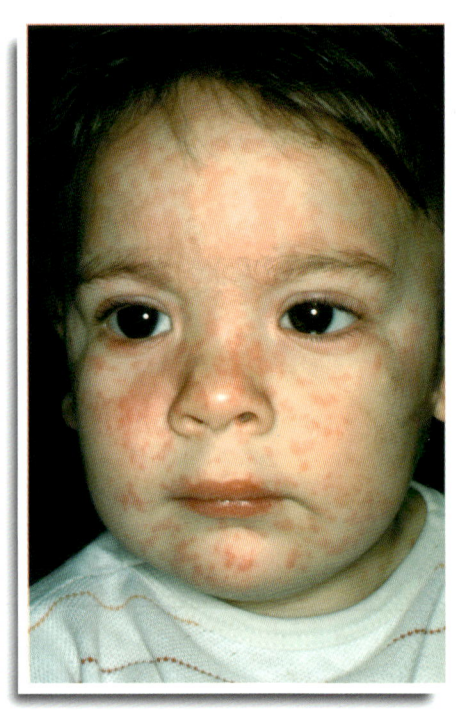

- One of childhood exanthemata due to RNA paramyxovirus with droplet / aerosol spread
- Incubation period 7 - 14 days, prodrome of fever, malaise, cough + conjunctivitis
- Small white (Koplik's spots) area in mouth adjacent to molars, like grains of salt on a red base
- Coincides with catarrhal prodrome, 24 - 48 hours later bright red erythema of forehead → whole face
- Rash becomes maculopapular → trunk + limbs. Resolution → brown discolouration + desquamation
- Contagious for 1 week after rash appears
- Complications - pneumonia, otitis media, encephalitis (rare)
- Reduces T cells → ↑ susceptibility to other infections e.g. TB
- Treatment: supportive + encourage high uptake of immunisation to maintain herd immunity

MELANOMA

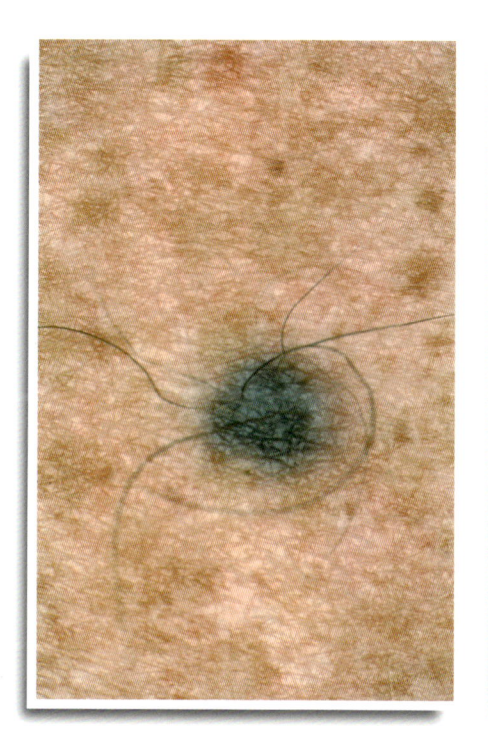

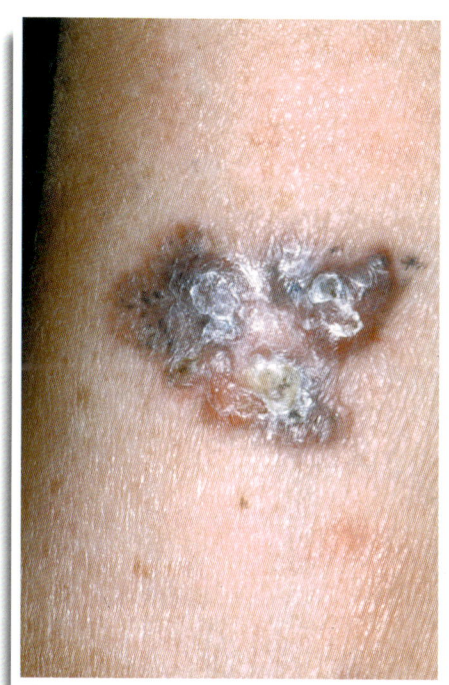

- An invasive malignant tumour of melanocytes, 30% arise within an existing mole
- Sun exposure major risk factor, commonest site - lower leg
- Occurs in fair complexion (primarily Celts) >30 years, Female >> Male
- Highly suspicious diagnosis if 2+ of the following features:
- A = asymmetry of lesion, periphery + surface
- B = irregularity of the border
- C = variation in colour
- D = diameter > 0.5cm
- E = elevation / enlargement also consider itching, bleeding, crusting

MELANOMA

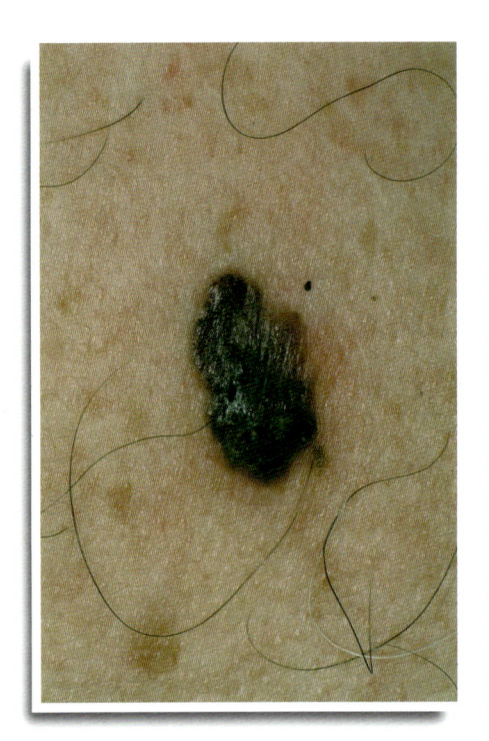

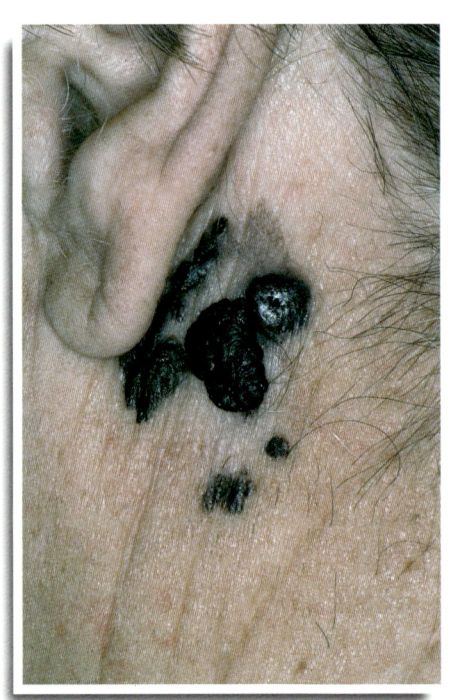

- Commonest clinical type: superficial spreading = early growth phase in horizontal direction
- Irregular surface contours + pigmentation with scalloped edge
- Nodular variety - less common but grows rapidly, often confused with benign mole
- Vertical growth of prime importance → invades blood vessels / lymphatic → metastases
- Prognosis related to depth of invasion (Breslow's thickness)
- 5 year survival: <1mm - 80-90%, > 3mm 40-50%
- Treatment: excision, 1-2 cm margin of normal skin. Lymph node involvement → block dissection
- Radiotherapy for: very large tumours, on head + neck if excision difficult, or recurrent skin metastases
- Lentigo Maligna (Hutchinson's Freckle) - premalignant intraepidermal pigmented macule -
- Irregular well defined border, slowly enlarging, middle age - elderly
- Risk of malignant change by 75 years = 1%. Treatment: local excision rather than cryotherapy

MENINGOCOCCAL RASH

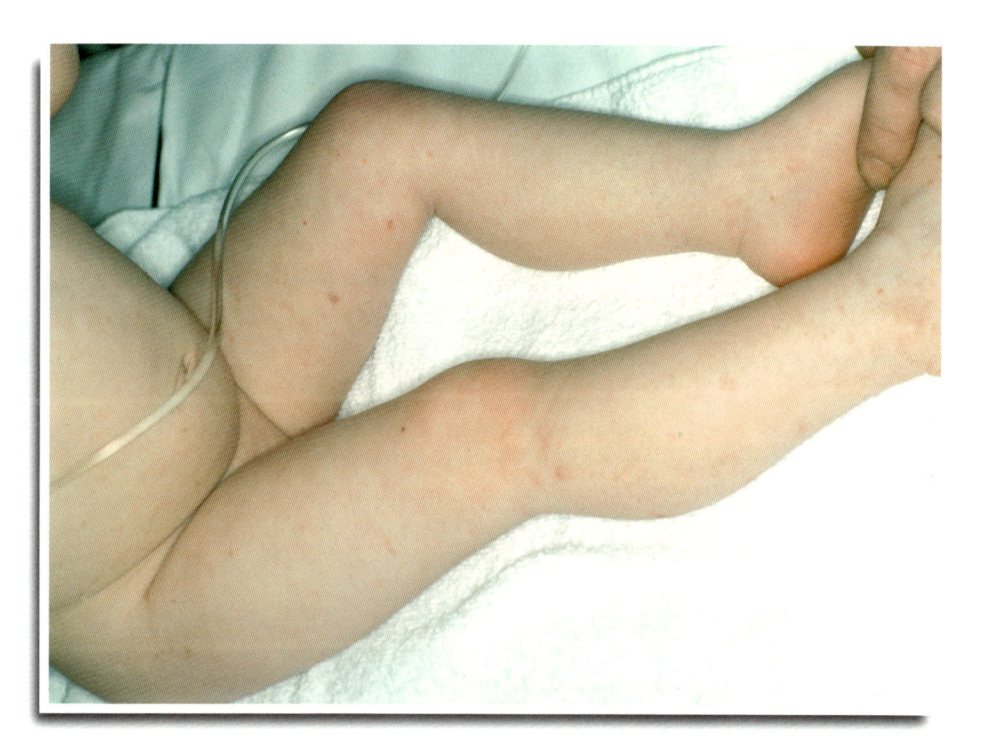

- Haemorrhagic + necrotic cutaneous lesions associated with Gram neg. N. Meningitides
- Any age primarily 1st decade. Droplet spread. Mid Winter / early Spring
- Short incubation → small purpuric papules / petechiae, often on legs with fever + meningism
- Bacteraemia → life threatening multi-organ involvement due to immune-complex vasculitis
- Can lead to intravascular coagulation + bacterial damage to blood vessels
- Treatment: high dose parental antibiotics at diagnosis - delay can be fatal
- Oral rifampicin / ciprofloxacin (not licensed) to contacts
- Vaccinate contacts in epidemics

METASTATIC NODULES

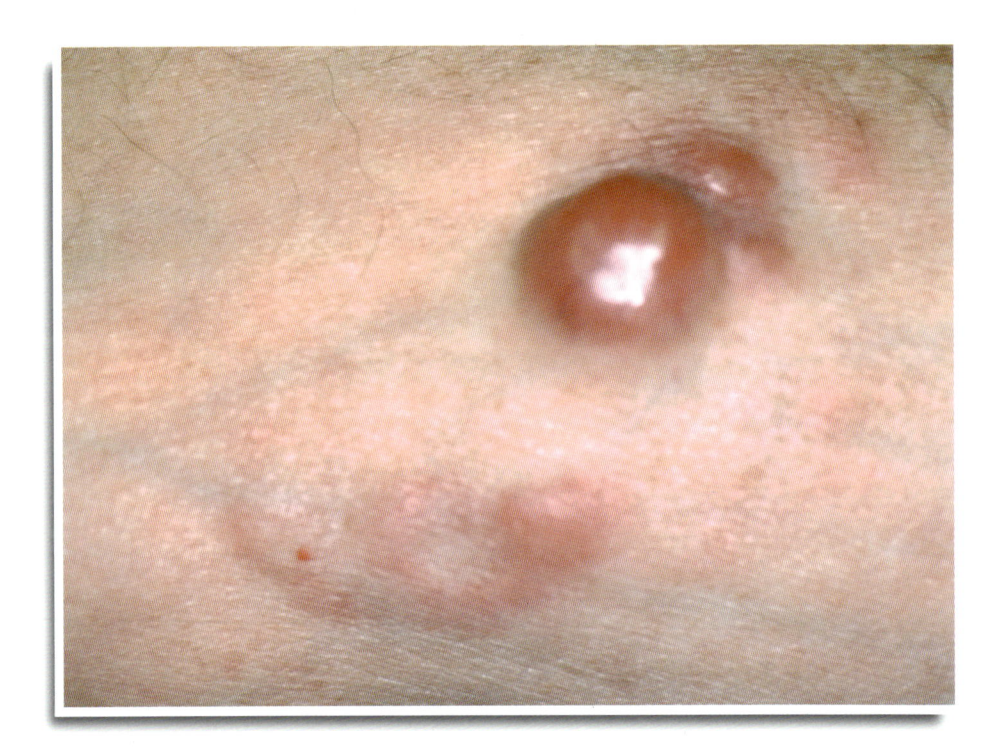

- Solitary / multiple dermal or subcutaneous nodules / papules / plaques
- Inflammatory, pink / red or blue / black, firm / indurated lesions or nodular lesions → ulcerate
- Represent deposition of cells from distant primary tumour (often presenting feature)
- Transported by blood / lymphatics / across peritoneal cavity
- Incidence: 0.7% - 9% of all patients with carcinoma, usually elderly,
- Female - primarily breast, colon, melanoma, lung + ovary
- Male - primarily lung, colon, melanoma, SCC mouth, kidney + stomach
- Patients with known carcinoma with skin mets = poor prognosis (approx. 3 months survival)
- Exception - contiguous spread of breast carcinoma, patient can survive for years
- Treatment: if solitary / few + patient not terminal → excise

MILIA

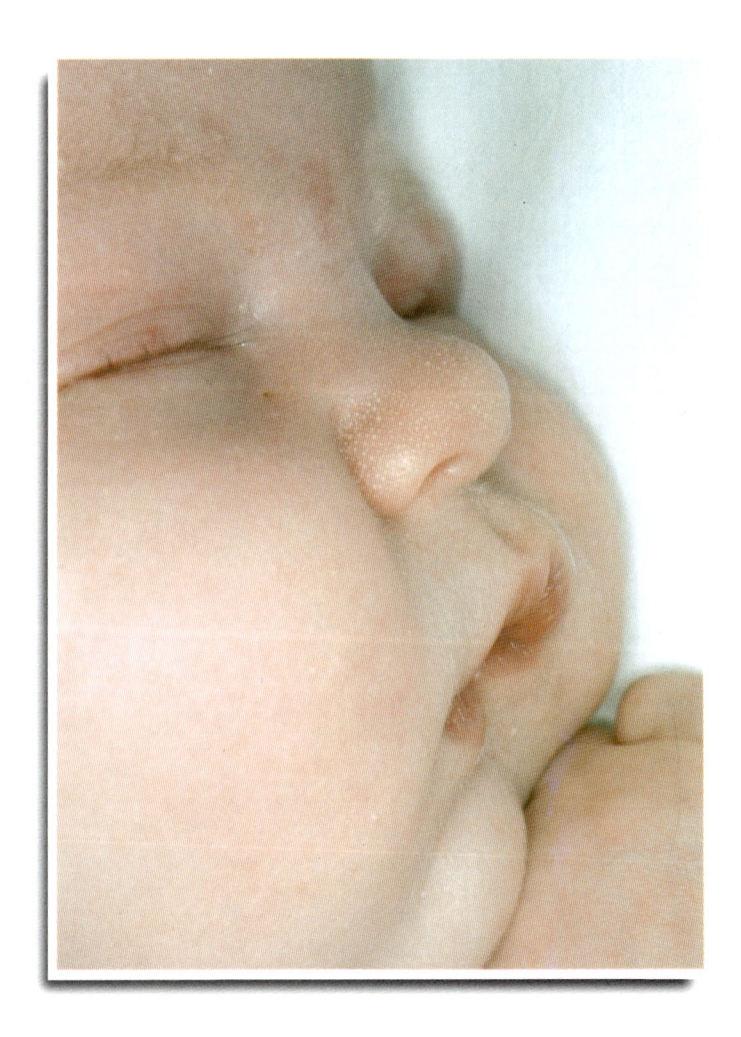

- Small sub-epidermal keratin cysts
- Tiny white "millet seed-like" papules 0.5 - 2 mm diameter under skin
- Common on face of all age groups, can appear after any blistering eruption
- In neonates due to retention of keratin + sebaceous material in pilosebaceous apparatus
- Eruptive form, arising from sweat ducts / hair follicles, around eyes in teenagers
- Resolves spontaneously in babies. Older individuals - contents can be picked out with needle

MOLE
"Melanocytic Naevus"

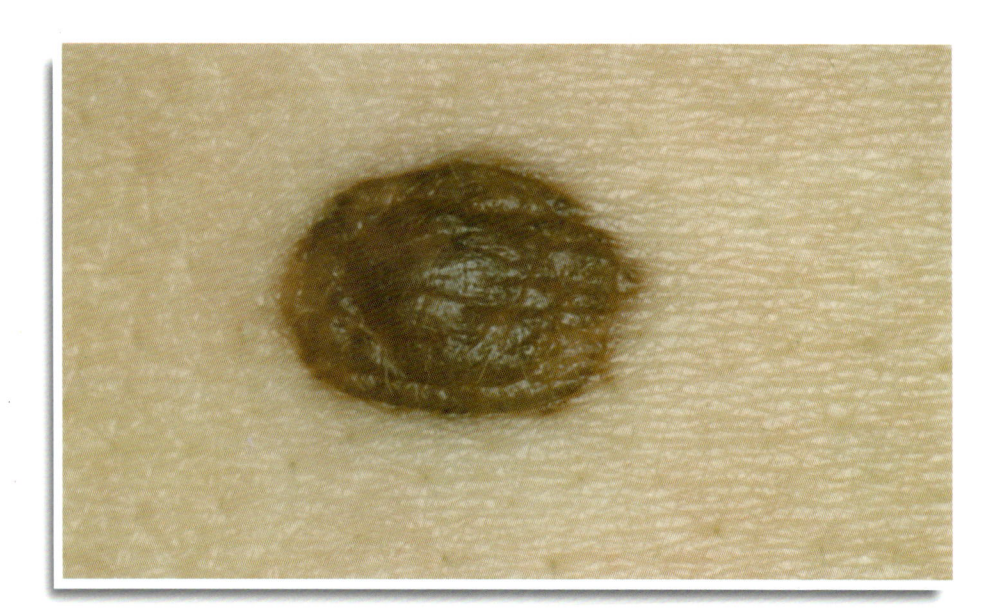

- Common, benign, pigmented lesions representing ↑ melanocytes in skin
- Classified as: Junctional / compound / intradermal, according to position of naevus cells in skin
- Uniform colour, even surface, static in size or very slow growing
- Arise in childhood / adolescence. Primarily Caucasian's on face, neck + back
- ↑ number of moles seen in pregnancy + oestrogen therapy
- Naevus matures → later degenerates → disappears, so less numerous in elderly
- Compound naevus most common: slightly raised / pigmented, tend to arise in older children
- Junctional + intradermal component, can be hair bearing
- Treatment: should protect from sun as small risk of malignant change
- Excise for cosmetic reasons only, preferably in teens / adulthood

MOLLUSCUM CONTAGIOSUM

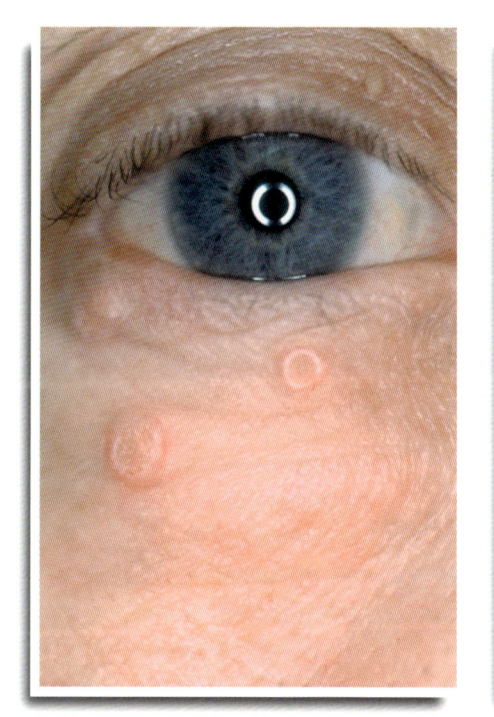

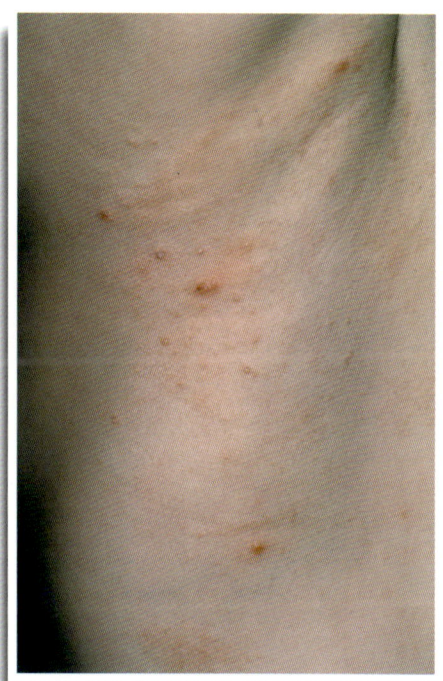

- DNA Pox virus infection of skin spread by direct contact
- Incubation 2 - 6 weeks. Children more common than adults, Male > Female
- 1 - 5 mm white / pink umbilicated papules with central keratotic plug (contains molluscum bodies)
- Primarily face, eyelids, neck, axillae, trunk + ano-genital area
- Single (often giant mollusca) or multiple (widespread in HIV, atopy, sarcoid + immuno-compromised)
- Lasts 6 - 9 months → spontaneous resolution due to cell mediated immunity
- Treatment: prick with sterile needle / orange stick dipped in phenol / weak iodine + express contents
- Cryotherapy helpful for larger lesions

MONGOLIAN BLUE SPOT

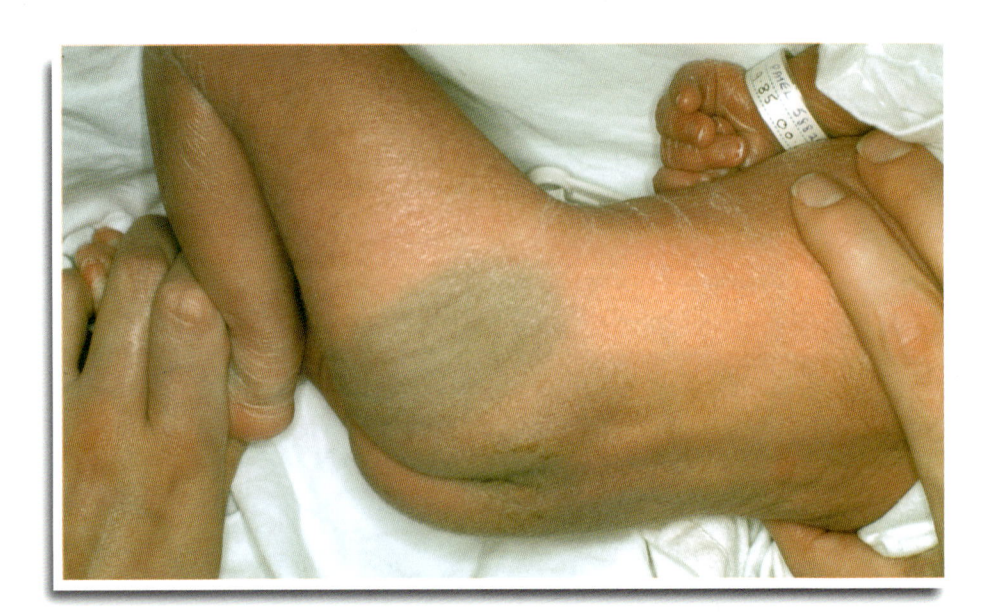

- Large, benign, pigmented macule primarily over lower back (can occur anywhere including face)
- Common in Oriental / Afro-Caribbean neonates (<10% Caucasians), present at birth
- Melanocytes deep in dermis → bruise-like appearance
- Usually single although can be multiple on trunk
- May darken in neonatal period, gradually fades / disappears in childhood
- Treatment: none. No malignant potential
- N.B. should not be mistaken for non-accidental injury

NAEVUS - COMPOUND MELANOCYTIC

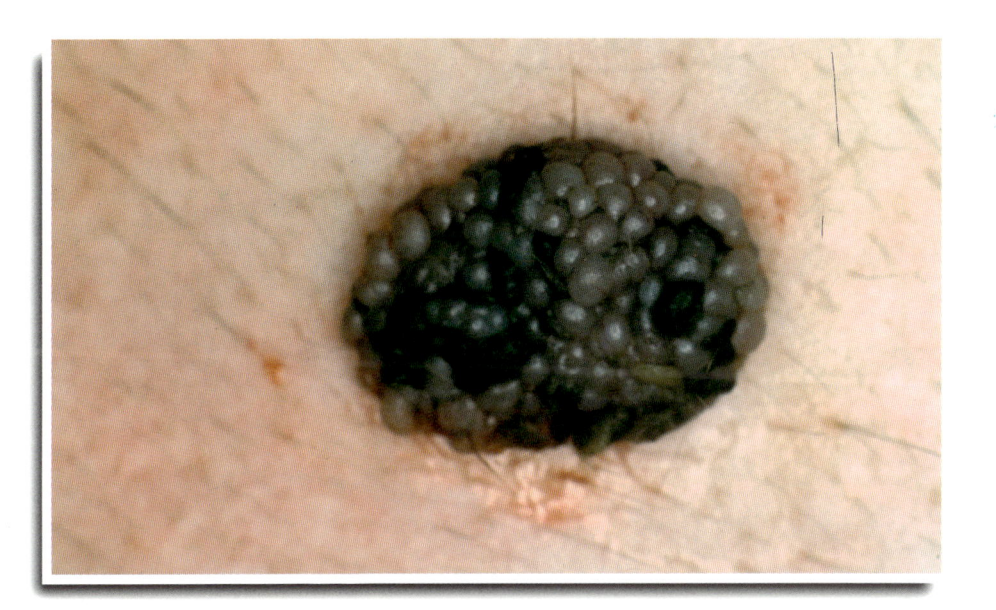

- Domed, pigmented nodules with light / dark brown, even colouration
- Can → large + smooth or with cerebriform / hyperkeratotic / papillomatous surface +/- hair
- Cells in dermis + junctional layer
- Natural history of a mole: Junctional Naevus (flat + brown) → Compound Naevus (brown papule) → Intradermal Naevus (skin coloured papule) - this represents normal benign change
- Once melanocytes migrate to dermis, malignant potential is lost

NAEVUS - CONGENITAL MELANOCYTIC

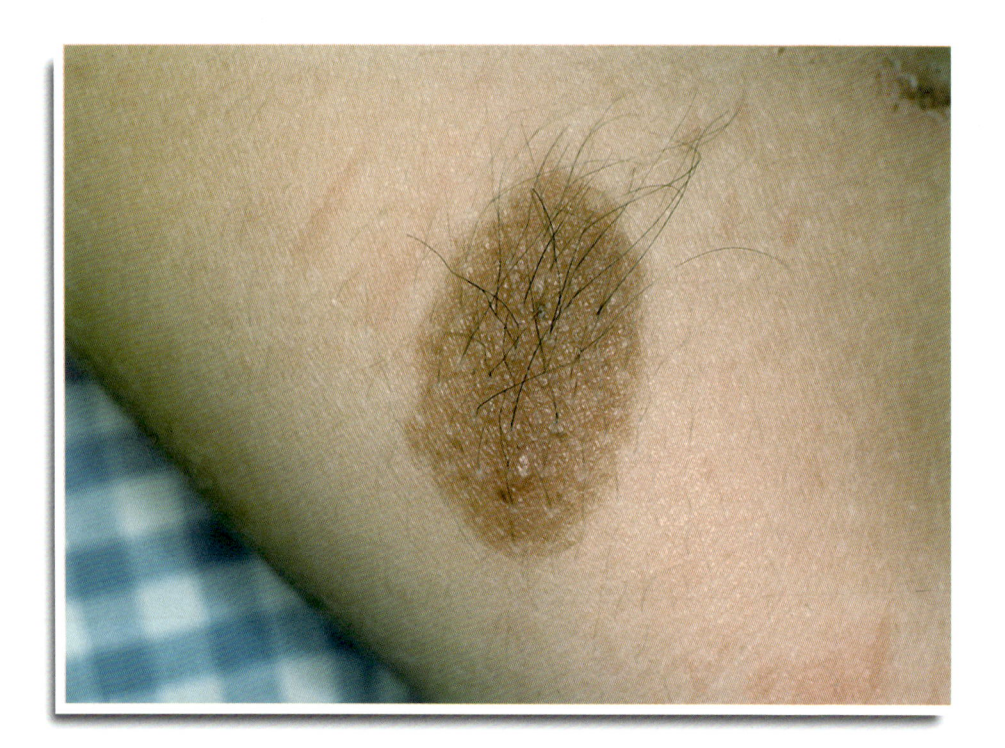

- Larger + more deeply pigmented than acquired naevi, may have coarse hairs
- May be red at birth + pigment within months → flat or raised / hairy or warty
- Male = Female, all races. 1% of white neonates, majority < 3 cm diameter
- Small risk of malignant change in larger lesions (>2 cm) in adult life
- Can persist → old age (unlike acquired naevi)
- Worst example: bathing trunk naevus - can occupy 50% body surface
- Treatment: monitor + report changes, some suggest elective removal of small lesions

NAEVUS - SEBACEOUS
"Sebaceous Naevus of Jadassohn / Organoid Naevus"

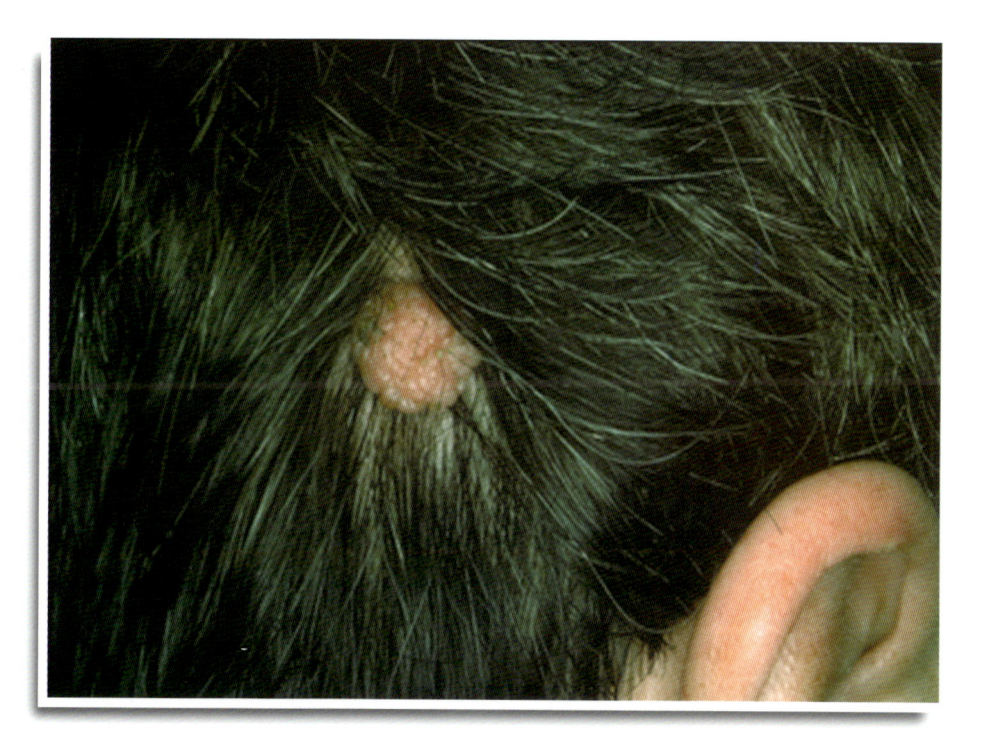

- Uncommon but important papillomatous hamartoma with epidermal + dermal elements
- Congenital - 3 : 1000 babies. Malformation of sebaceous differentiation on scalp (rarely face)
- Hairless, warty, thin (linear or oval), elevated, 1 - 2 cm orange plaque
- 10% can → BCC primarily in 4th decade
- Multiple lesions = epidermal naevus syndrome / Jadassohn's phakomatosis → Associated with neurological / developmental defects + high incidence of internal malignancy
- Treatment: excise at puberty for cosmetic reasons + to pre-empt malignant change

NAEVUS - SPILUS

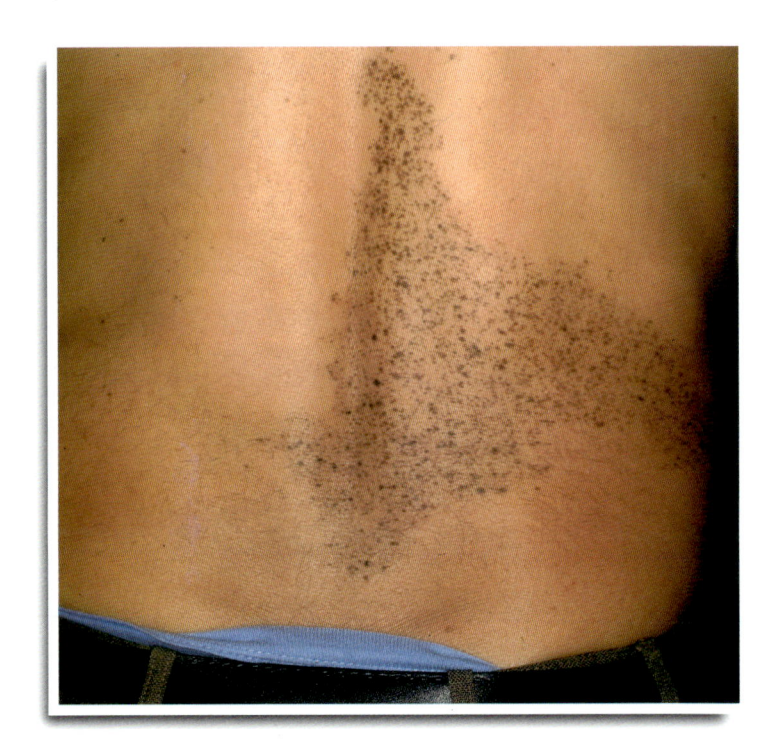

- Latin: spilus = spot. Relatively rare birthmark
- Dark speckled macules / papules within larger pigmented patch
- ↑ melanocytes in back ground pigmentation + lentiginous melanocytic hyperplasia in darker spots
- Lesions often large + occasionally associated with neurofibromatosis
- Very rarely malignant change can occur → malignant melanoma
- Treatment: ? advise prophylactic excision if lesion not too large

NECROBIOSIS LIPOIDICA DIABETICORUM

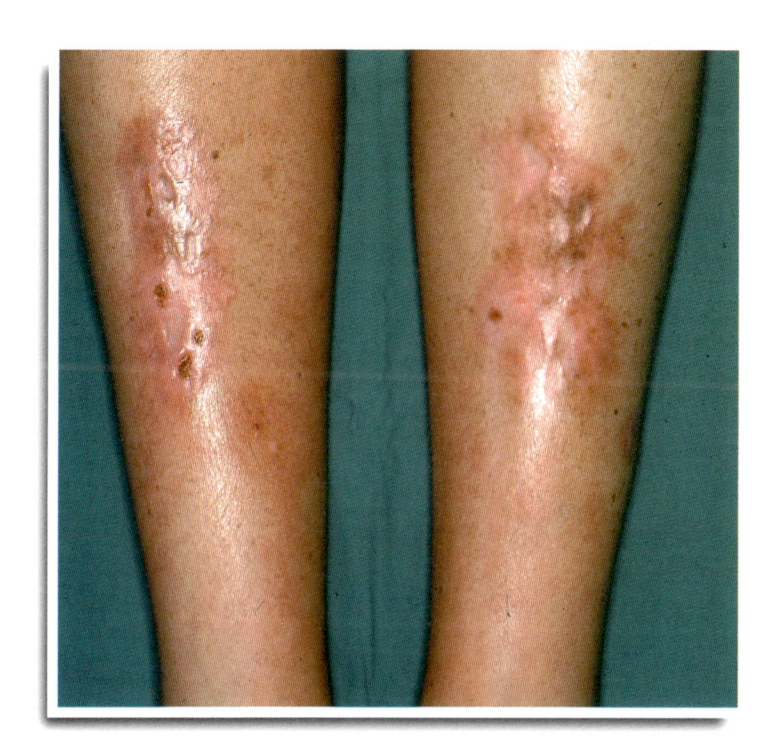

- Shiny, atrophic skin lesion primarily on shins (>80%). Seen in < 1% diabetics
- 1/3 patients have diabetes, 1/3 might develop diabetes & 1/3 never will
- Extent of lesions not related to severity of diabetes, improving diabetic control has no effect
- Primarily teens / young adults, Male : Female 3 : 1
- Circumscribed plaques, irregular pink / yellow surface. Persists for long periods
- Margin - violet / erythematous, underlying blood vessels visible through atrophic skin
- Degenerative collagen fibres replaced by lipid ?due to micro-angiopathy
- Often seen in association with granuloma annulare
- Treatment: resistant to all forms of therapy, intralesional Triamcinolone can prevent enlargement
- Potent steroids with occlusion helpful but some will ulcerate due to this therapy
- Minor trauma (including biopsy) can → ulceration

ONYCHOMYCOSIS
Tinea Unguium

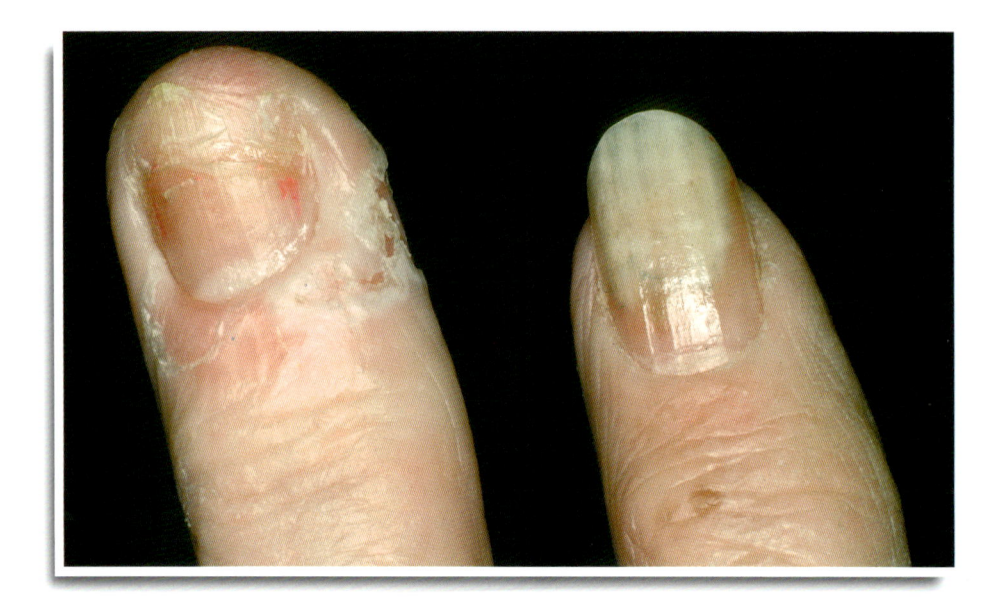

- Infection of nail due to fungi / yeasts / moulds, 20 - 50 year olds
- Primary onychomycosis involves healthy nail, secondary involves diseased / traumatised nail
- Course of infection: discolouration → distal subungual hyperkeratosis → onycholysis
- Nail bed + fold often spared with dermatophyte infection
- Candida invades proximal nail fold → paronychia, nail plate involvement → dystrophy
- Aggravating factors: wet environment, occlusive footwear, communal bathing + poor arterial circulation
- Source of infection: dermatophytes (Tinea Unguium) - direct contact with patient / fomites
- Candida - normal flora → problematic if local conditions encourage yeasts or immuno-compromised
- Moulds - environmental (often soil) with no human - human transmission
- In children often due to cross infection from adult with tinea pedis
- Treatment: nail parings from under surface of nail to confirm diagnosis
- Oral antifungals - fewer relapses with newer agents, topical therapy less effective

quick reference atlas of dermatology

PALMAR ERYTHEMA

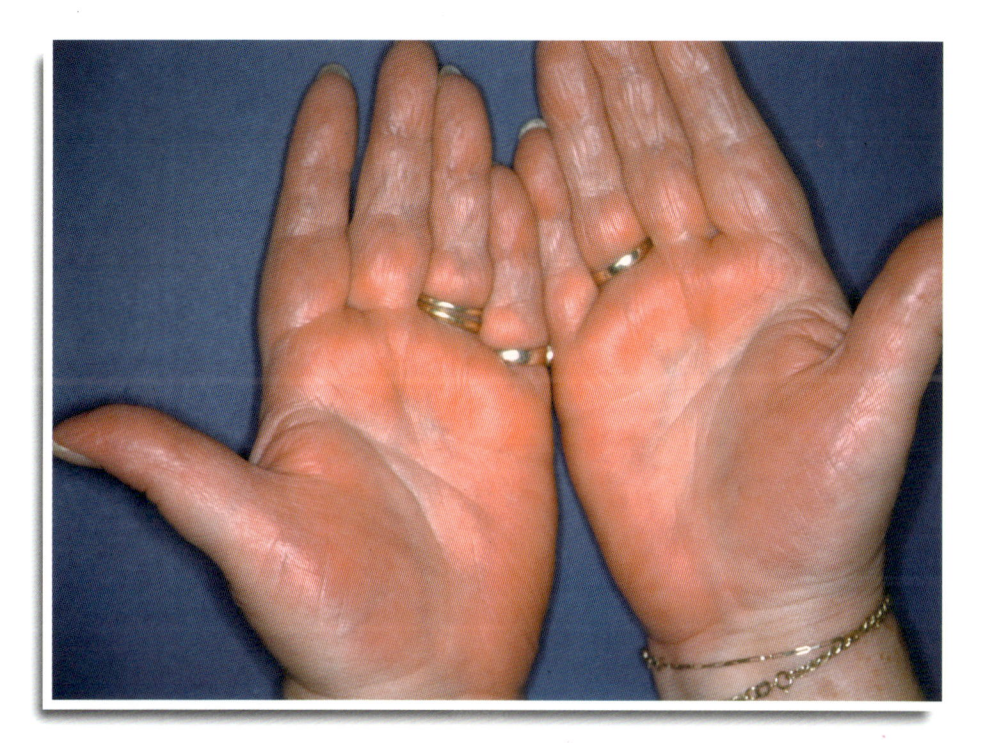

- Can occur in isolation in normal patient + in familial cases
- Associated with pregnancy, liver disease & rheumatoid arthritis
- Often seen with spider naevi, may be due to increased circulating oestrogens
- Treatment: none unless secondary cause can be identified

PARONYCHIA

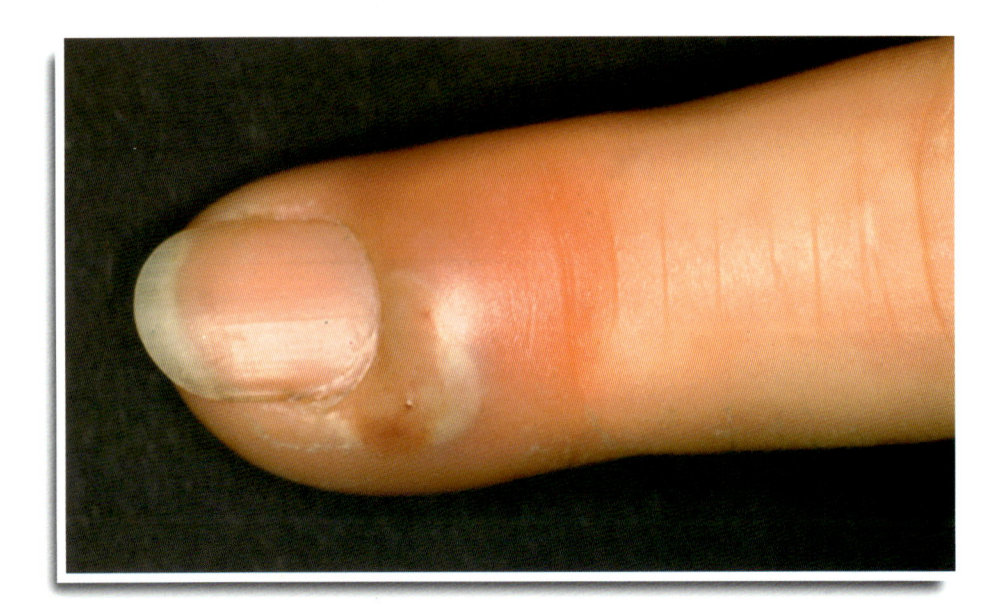

- Acute + chronic, painful, pustular infection of nail fold
- Acute: Staph' > Strep' → painful red swelling with pus formation
- Rarely H. Simplex infection but vesicles would be evident
- Chronic: Gram +ve cocci / Gram -ve rods / Candida Albicans
- Cuticle lost due to trauma / excess water immersion. Less swelling, dull red + no pus formation
- Swelling → pressure on nail plate → longitudinal nail ridging
- Secondary invasion with bacteria often seen e.g. Pseudomonas → green discolouration
- Predisposing factors: water / trauma / poor peripheral circulation / diabetes
- Primarily adults or thumb sucking children, nail polish users + food handlers
- Treatment: if no pus visible → oral antibiotics
- Obvious pus → incision + drainage, keep hands dry to allow new cuticle growth (3 - 4 months)
- Protective film of petroleum jelly several times per day helpful

PEMPHIGOID - BULLOUS

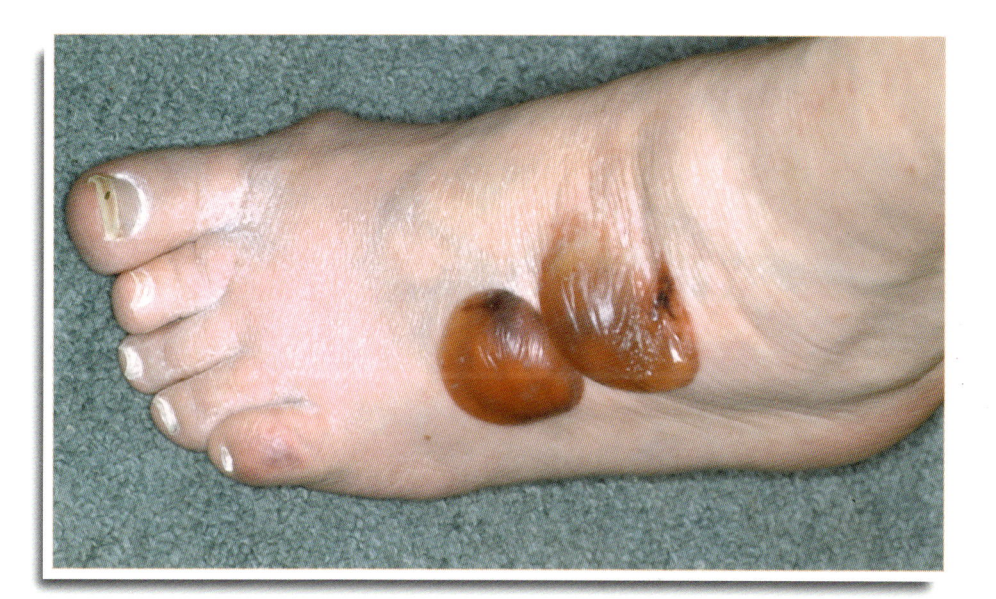

- Disease of elderly (60 - 80 years) Male = Female
- Autoimmune disease with IgG antibodies at epidermis / dermis junction
- Tense, blood filled bullae appear rapidly over preceding urticarial / erythematous rash → normal skin
- Primarily trunk + flexural aspects of limbs, sometimes itchy, no associated fever / malaise
- Occasionally blisters seen in mouth → erosions
- Bullae are subepidermal + persistent, remission occurs after many months
- Localised type affecting legs of elderly Female runs benign self limiting course
- In a minority of cases it is a skin marker of neoplasia
- Treatment: initial high dose oral steroids (40 - 60 mg Prednisolone) → reduce with time
- Azothiaprine improves remission rate / ↓ steroid dose
- Topical steroids can be used on early / developing lesions
- Treatment can last 1 - 2 years (death can result from fluid loss or fatal steroid effects)

PEMPHIGUS VULGARIS

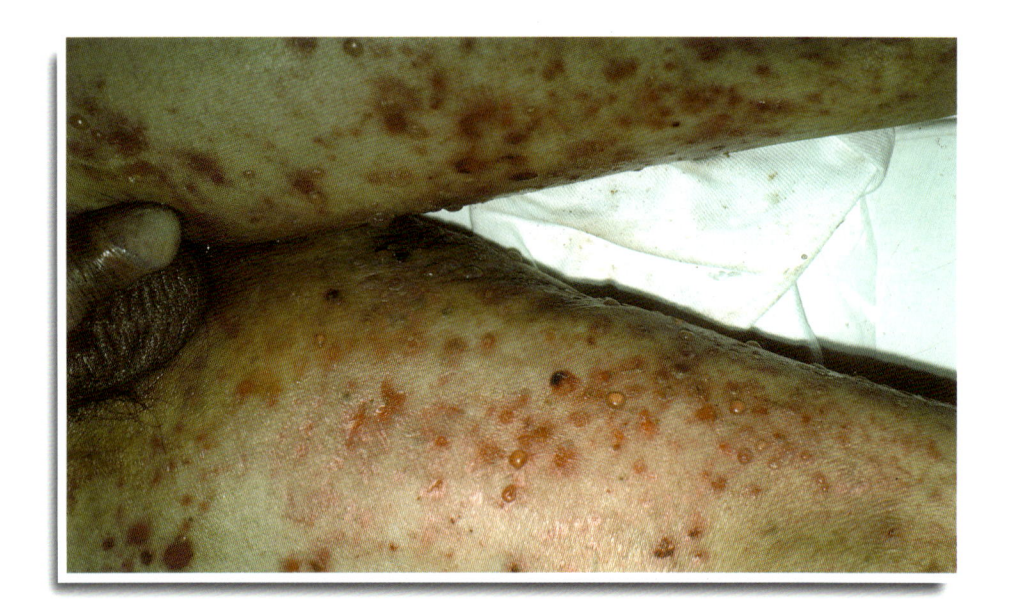

- Uncommon, autoimmune condition (antigen unknown), age: 40 - 60 years, Male = Female
- Individual epidermal cells separate from each other → superficial blistering
- Blisters rupture → erosions → crusts. Never haemorrhagic (unlike pemphigoid) + not irritant
- Rubbing normal skin → sloughing of epidermis (Nikolsky sign)
- Erosions appear in mouth weeks / months before skin lesions appear (scalp, face, trunk + flexures)
- Rapid spread can lead to death due to fluid loss and secondary infection
- Treatment: very high dose steroids (80 - 320 mg prednisolone daily) ↓ dose to maintenance level
- Potassium permanganate in bath to dry blisters
- Azothiaprine useful if steroids not controlling the blistering, methotrexate, gold + plasmaphoresis
- When apparently disease free for 3 months and antibody (IgG) negative - therapy stops
- Side effects of therapy are the commonest cause of death

PITYRIASIS ROSEA

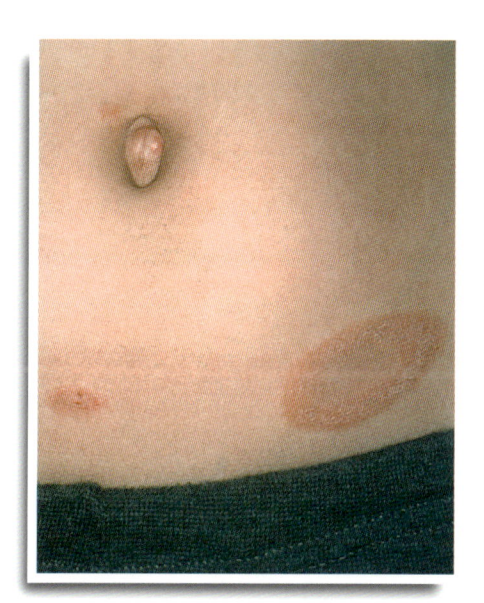

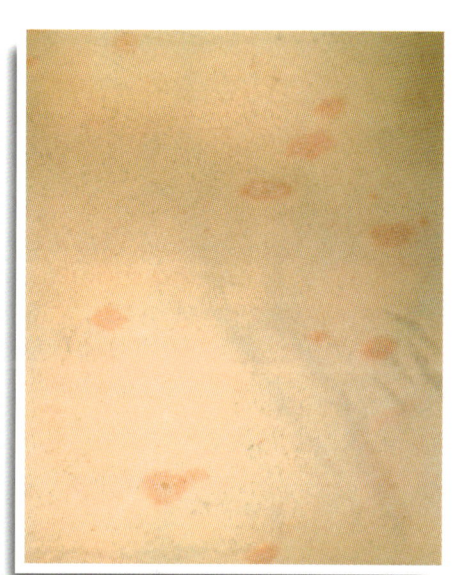

- Rash in fit, healthy children / young adults. Peak incidence Spring + Autumn
- Cause unknown (probably viral) + not contagious
- Single, oval, scaling plaque, 2 - 3 cm diameter, appears on trunk / limb = herald patch
- Few days later small, pink, follicular papules or petaloid lesions appear (smaller than herald patch)
- If herald patch on trunk → rash on vest / pant area. Lesions follows Langer's lines (Xmas tree pattern)
- If herald patch on limb → rash on limbs, if on neck → rash on face + trunk
- No associated ill health or other symptoms
- Lasts 2 - 10 weeks → spontaneous resolution → slight pigmentation → fading
- N.B. secondary syphilis can mimic this condition - if unwell with rash do VDRL test
- Pityriasis rosea-like rash seen with gold, captopril, barbiturates + penicillamine
- Treatment: none. Sun exposure helpful. Calamine + mild steroid creams if itchy

PITYRIASIS VERSICOLOR

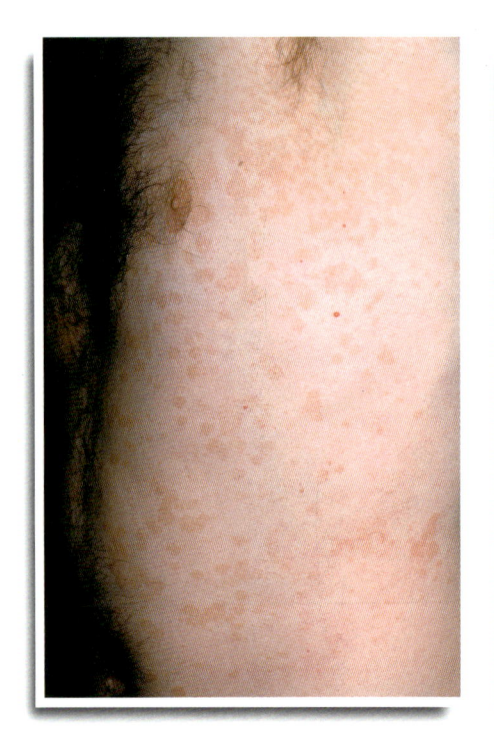

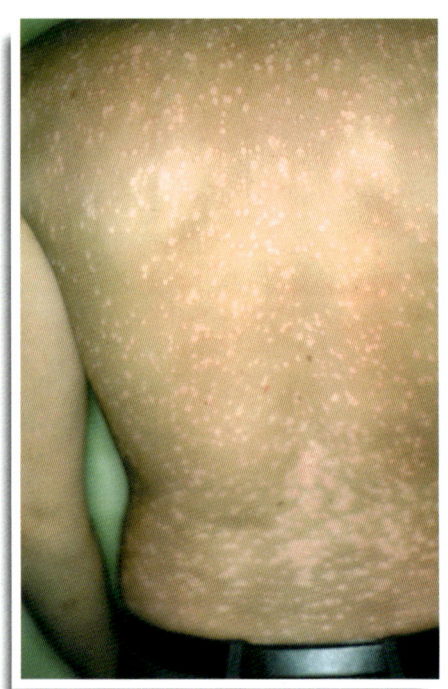

- Pityriasis = bran like. Versicolor = variable colour
- Non contagious, superficial yeast infection primarily of trunk, can → temporary hypopigmentation
- Adults + adolescents (5% cases are in children when it can involve the face)
- Pityrosporum ovale is normal commensal in hair follicles
- Becomes a pathogen if ↑ humidity at skin surface +/or ↑ sebum production
- Multiple fawn / pinkish brown patches → plaques with well defined border
- Pale patches on tanned skin, brown patches on covered skin
- Diagnosis: scrapings show short, branched hyphae + spores (spaghetti + meatballs)
- Treatment: Selenium Sulphide shampoo overnight → wash off + apply twice weekly for 3 weeks
- Alternative Ketoconzaole cream twice daily for 2 weeks or oral antifungal agents
- Recurrence is common

POMPHOLYX
"Vesicular Palmar Eczema / Dyshidrotic Eczema"

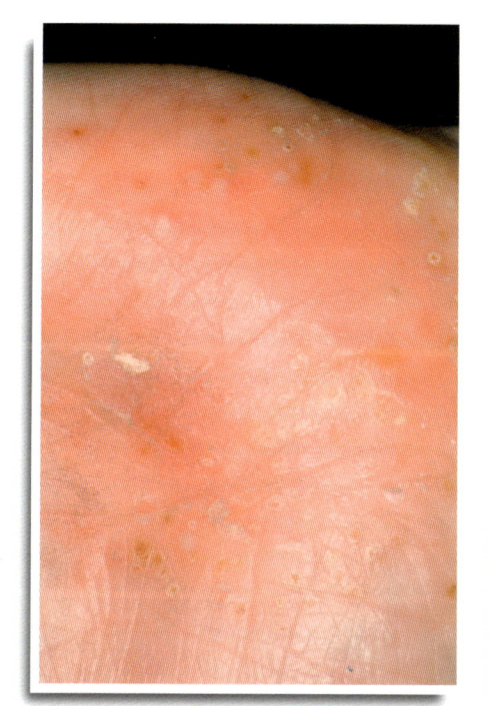

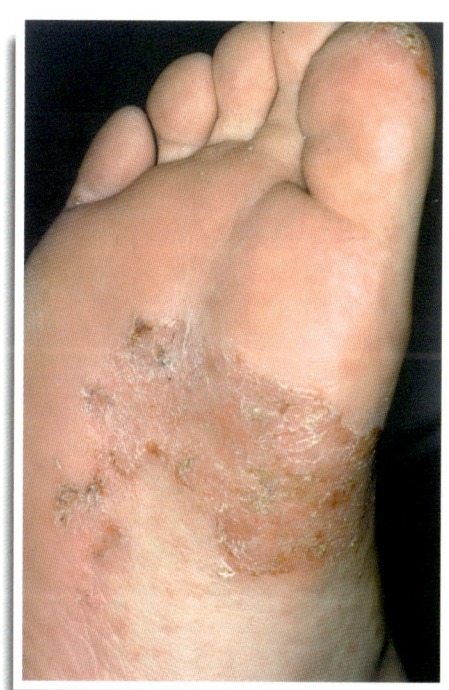

- Vesicular type of hand (80%) and foot dermatitis, age 12 - 40 years, Male = Female
- Acute / chronic / recurrent, deep seated, itchy "tapioca like" vesicles → coalesce → bullae
- Scaling → fissuring → lichenification + desquamation. Can become secondarily infected
- Lasts several weeks, can be recurrent with considerable nuisance factor
- 50% patients are atopic, aggravating factors: emotional stress, hot / humid conditions
- Hyperhidrosis can be associated but no sweat gland dysfunction per se
- Treatment: puncture (do not de-roof) large bullae, Potassium Permanganate soaks to dry lesions
- Topical steroids (+/- occlusion) for 2 weeks, antibiotics for secondary infection

PSORIASIS

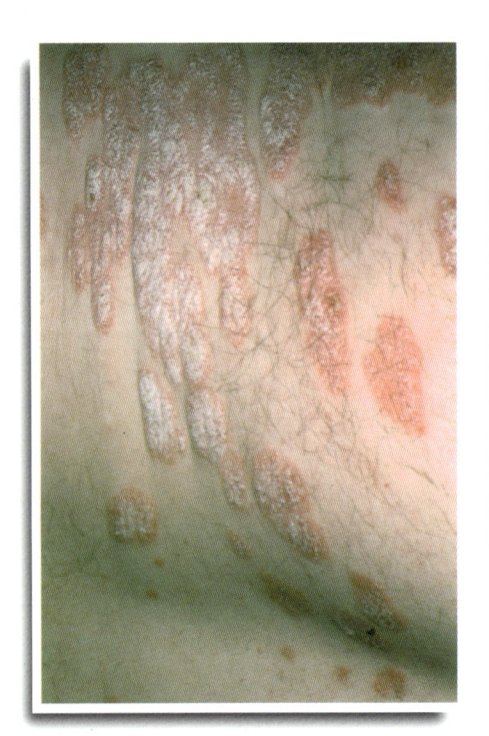

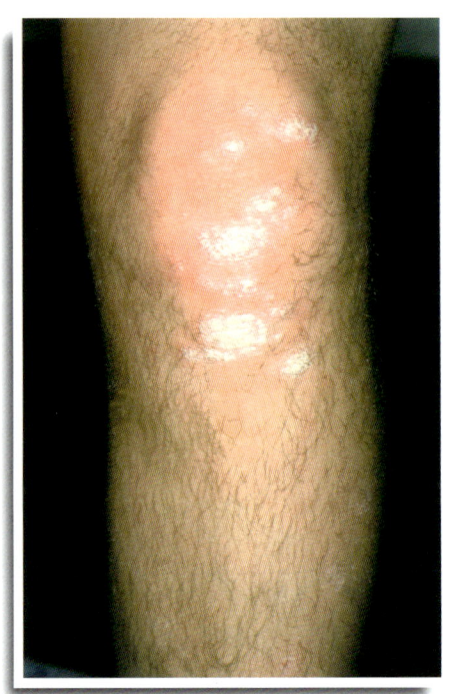

- Chronic, non infectious condition with hyper-proliferation of epidermis + high cell turnover
- Affects 1.5 - 2% population, any age but primarily 15 - 40 years, Male = Female
- Rare under age 10 years (then Female > Male), if < 2 years old, presents as napkin psoriasis
- Hereditary autosomal dominant with variable penetrance (1 parent affected - 25% chance)
- Trigger factors: trauma (Koebner's phenomenon), sunlight (10%), emotional stress (40%+)
- Also drugs - systemic steroids, Lithium, antimalarials, Beta-blockers + possibly alcohol

PSORIASIS - PLAQUE

- Commonest presentation. Sharply demarcated papules / plaques with silvery / white scales
- Removal of scale → blood droplets (Auspitz phenomenon)
- Salmon pink plaques are round / oval / annular or linear
- Either single, localised multiple lesions or generalised, often spares exposed areas e.g. face
- Associated nail dystrophy + seronegative arthritis affecting single large joint
- Treatment: topical steroids, Vitamin D3 analogues (calcipotriol), PUVA, methotrexate + cyclosporin

PSORIASIS - FLEXURAL

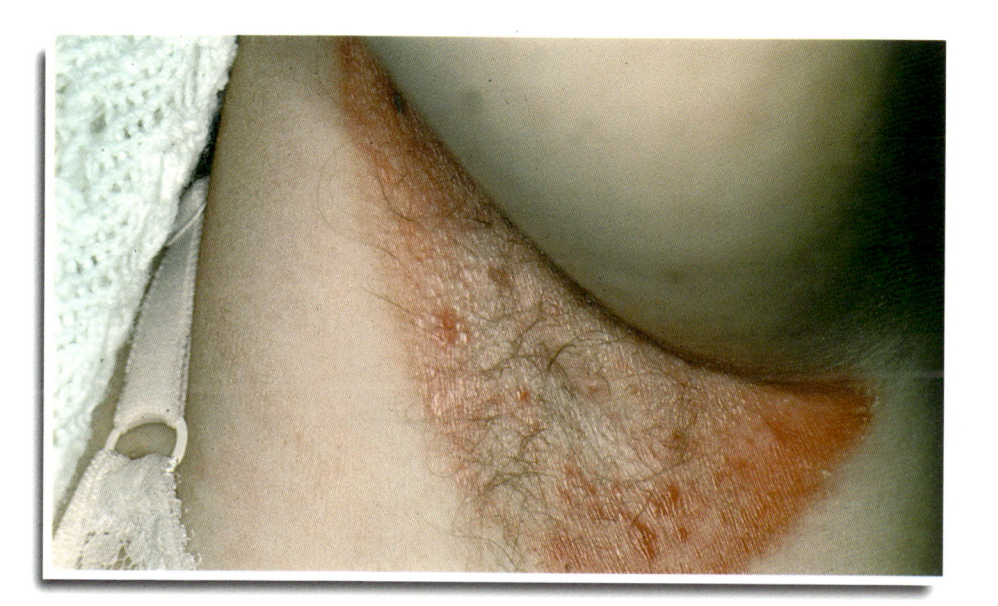

- Non scaling psoriasis of sub mammary / axillary / anogenital folds (scaling may occur at plaque edge)
- Glistening, sharply demarcated, erythematous plaques, can fissure in the depth of the fold
- Commonly mistaken for - candidiasis / tinea / intertrigo
- Often psoriasis present elsewhere. Commonest in Females + elderly
- Treatment: very vulnerable to steroid induced skin atrophy , use low potency steroid creams
- Calcipotriol is more effective + no risk of skin atrophy or tachyphylaxis

PSORIASIS - PUSTULAR

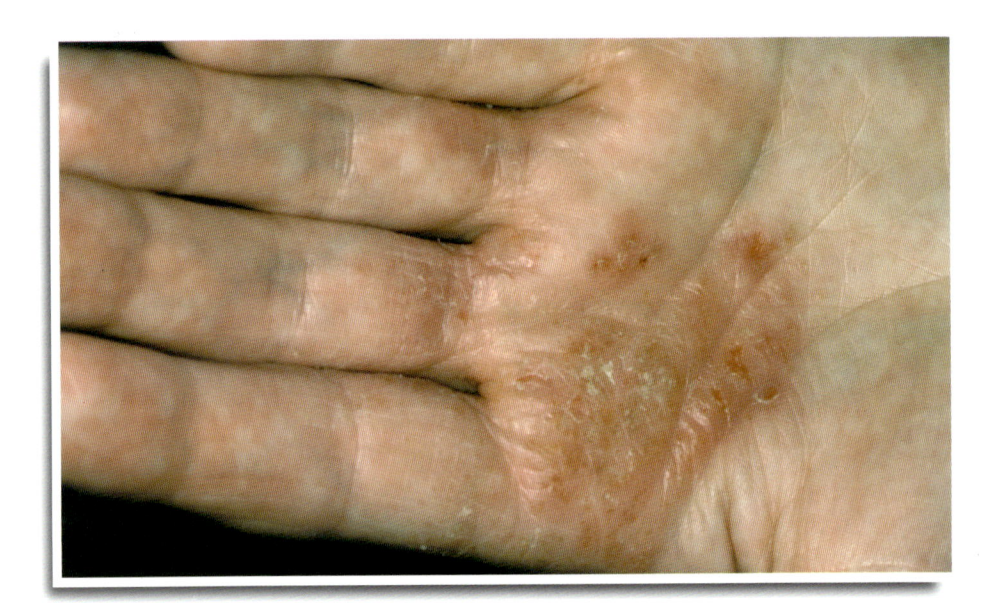

- Rare, chronic + relapsing condition (cause unknown), painful + difficult to treat
- Affects 50 - 60 year olds, Female : Male 4 : 1
- Palms + soles studded with numerous, sterile, 3 - 10 mm diameter pustules on erythematous base
- Always different coloured pustules visible representing different stages of development
- Pustules → brown macules or scales. Fissuring → extreme pain
- Von Zumbusch's disease: generalised eruption primarily in children, runs more benign course, possibly → plaque psoriasis in adulthood
- Treatment: moderate potent steroids + emollients, Methotrexate + PUVA if severe

PSORIASIS - SCALP

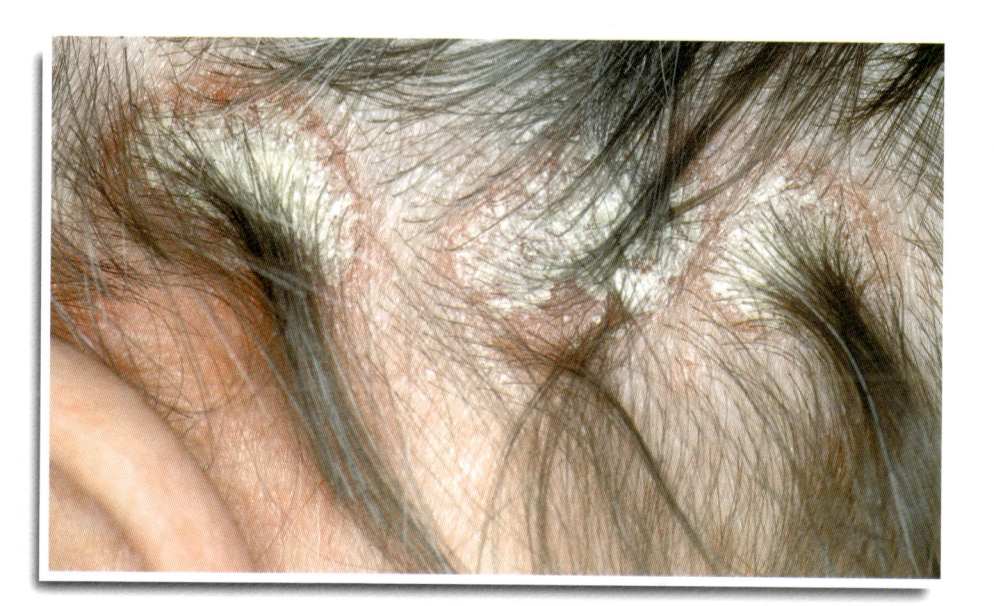

- Common, often first presenting site; discrete, red, itchy, scaly plaques which are palpable
- Often overflows beyond scalp margin → areas of scaling adjacent to normal skin
- Significant hair loss rare but thick scale removal can → associated hair loss
- Scales can grow out along the hairs (Pityriasis amantacea)
- Treatment: difficult + often resistant. Sunlight / PUVA of no help
- Resist scratching at all costs. Steroid / calcipotriol lotions very effective
- Salicylic acid + tar or oily (coconut) preparations containing Salicylic acid useful

PYODERMA GANGRENOSUM

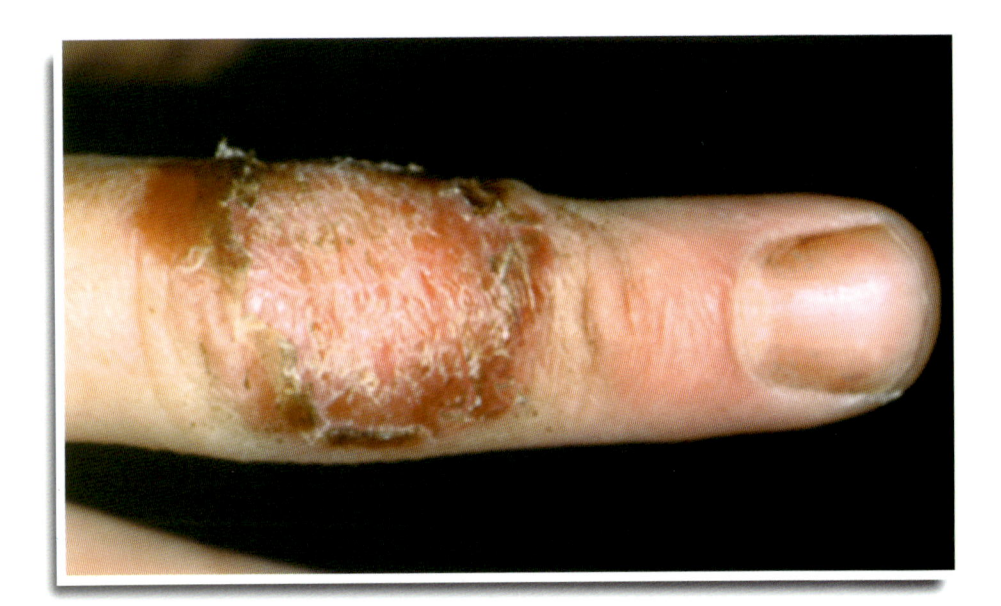

- Uncommon condition - large, single or multiple, rapidly spreading ulcers
- Inflamed nodule → painful necrotising ulceration with yellow honeycomb-like base
- Circular or polycyclic with blue, indurated / undermined or pustular margin
- Associated with: rheumatoid arthritis, inflammatory bowel disease or blood dyscrasias
- Prime sites: limbs > buttocks > abdomen > face.
- Probable immunological pathogenesis - a vasculitic process
- May arise in absence of underlying disease, can be caused by trauma e.g. biopsy + needle stick sites
- Can have fever + joint pain in acute stage, rarely aphthous stomatitis + ulceration mouth / conjunctivae
- Treatment: seek + treat underlying disease e.g. control of IBD → control of pyoderma
- Systemic steroids (dapsone in children), cyclosporin if steroid resistant
- Minocycline in older patients with subacute condition. Lesions heal → papery scars

PYOGENIC GRANULOMA
"Granuloma Telangiectaticum"

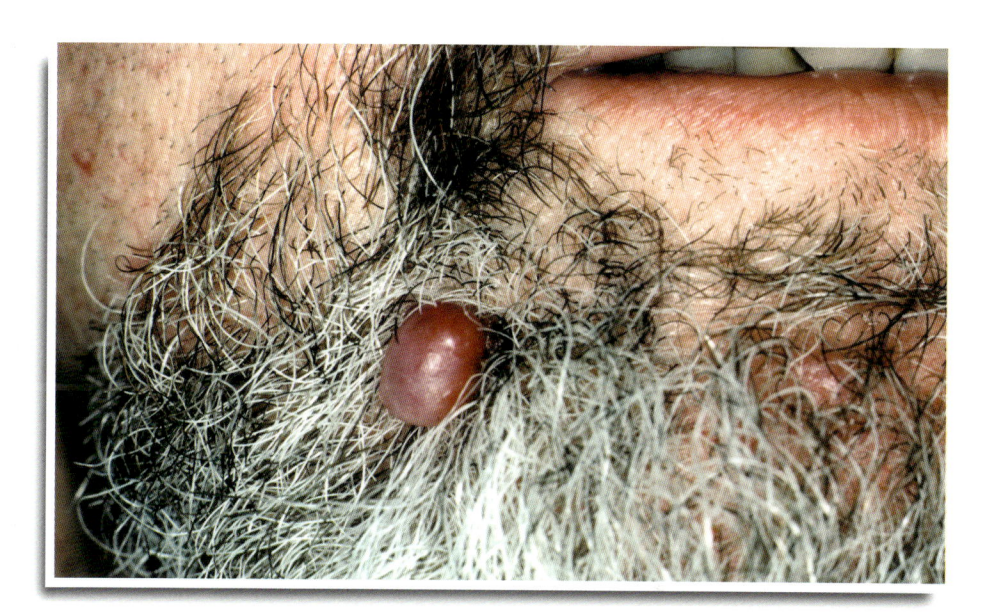

- Common, benign, acquired haemangioma due to trauma. Not granulomatous or pus forming
- Affects children, young adults. Male = Female
- Trauma → bright red, raised, pedunculated, raspberry-like lesion which develops over weeks
- Surrounding skin either normal or white thickened collarette present
- Bleeds very easily + surface can erode + crust
- Treatment: remove by curettage under local anaesthetic with cautery to base
- Note - treatment can → recurrence with satellites
- Can be confused with amelanotic melanoma hence → histology

ROSEOLA INFANTUM
"Exanthem Subitum"

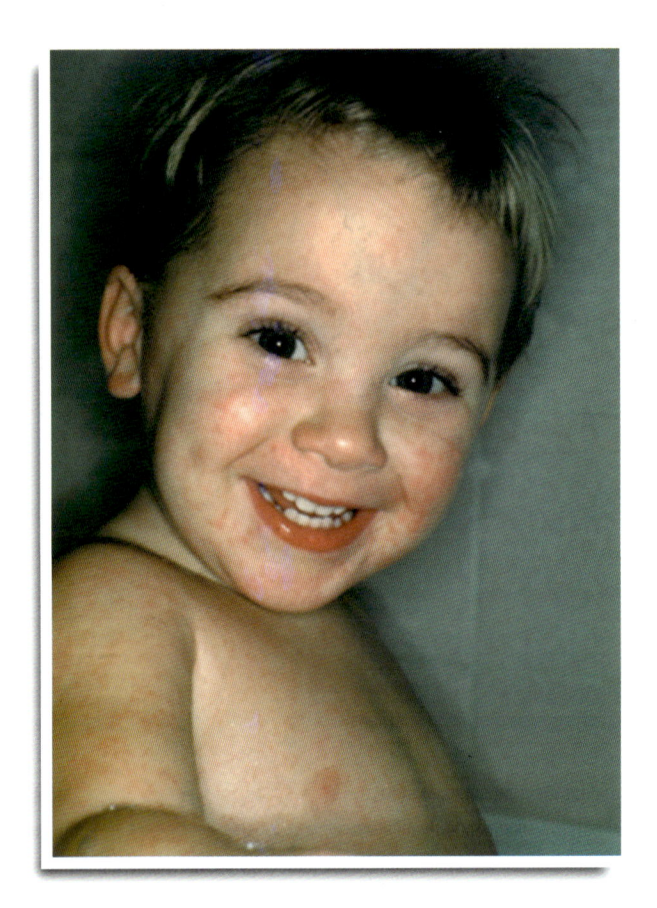

- Infectious viral disease (DNA human Herpes virus 6 & 7),
- Primarily 6 - 18 months old, 75% have antibodies by 1 year old
- Mild condition with virtually no malaise / systemic upset
- ↑ temp → ↓ temp → rash appears → persists over 2 - 4 days
- Multiple, pale pink, 1 - 5 mm macules / papules on neck + trunk, reticular pattern like rubella
- Complications: febrile convulsions, occipital lymphadenopathy
- Treatment: symptomatic only

RUBELLA
"German Measles / Three Day Measles"

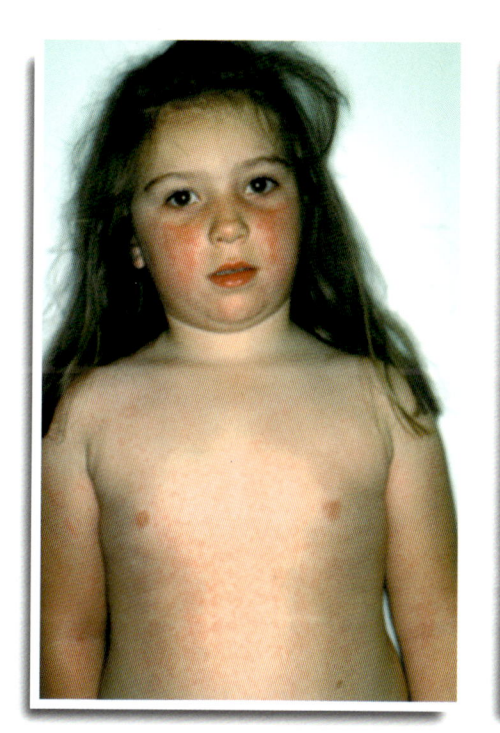

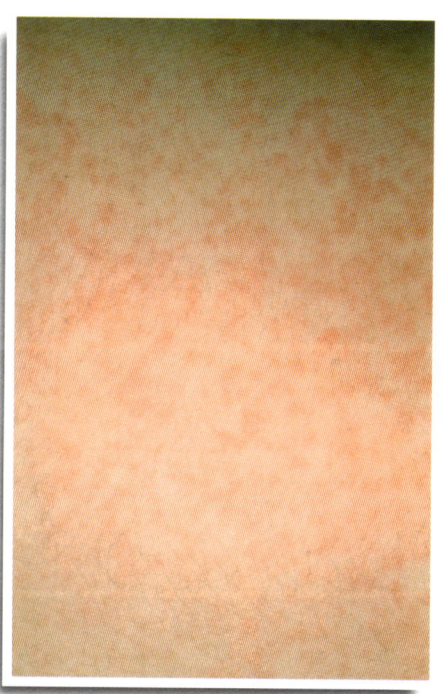

- Typically childhood exanthema due to RNA Togavirus, less common in young adults
- Droplet spread, 14 - 21 day incubation, often no prodrome except mild fever → rash appears
- Pale pink macules (face), caudal spread → confluent → fading (remains infectious for further 5 days)
- Associated features: tender occipital nodes / erythema of palate / arthritis in immunised adult Females
- Post auricular + post cervical nodes can persist for months
- Complications: splenic enlargement + generalised lymphadenopathy,
- Congenital defects if infection in 1st trimester (congenital rubella syndrome)
- Treatment: symptomatic only, if in doubt test rubella antibody titres
- Encourage routine immunisation

SCABIES

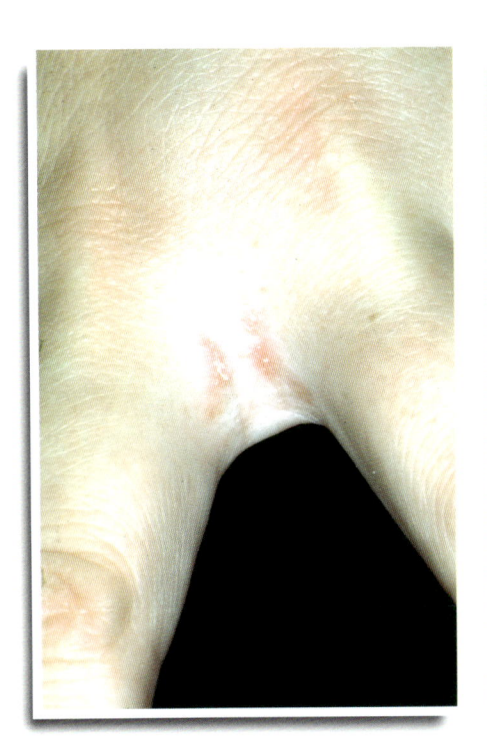

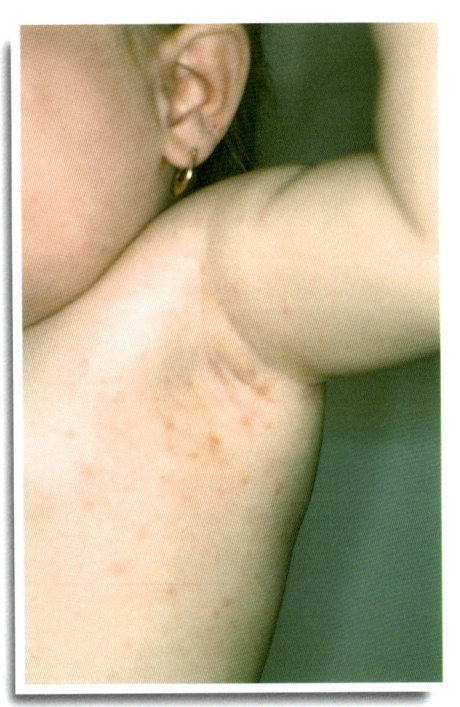

- Pruritic, very contagious infestation due to Sarcoptes Scabiei Var Hominis (usually <20 mites)
- Hallmark: serpiginous track = burrow in which female mite lays eggs
- Burrows primarily seen on soles, wrists, inter-digital spaces + genitalia (animal scabies - no burrows)
- Rash = Erythematous papules / pustules with excoriation ++
- Rash primarily seen on - fingers, wrists, nipples, abdomen, genitals, buttocks + ankles
- Large, inflammatory, rubbery lesions can develop on scrotum, elbows + axillae
- These can occasionally be widespread + last up to 1 year
- Primarily children affected (rash widely disseminated + often vesicular), spread by close contact
- Incubation = 1 month → insidious itch → intense when hot (due to sensitisation to mite + eggs)
- Complication - Norwegian scabies - crusted eruption due to thousands of mites → "7 year itch"
- Treatment: appropriate topical scabicides, including all close contacts, hot wash clothes / bedding
- Relapses common, re-infestation → itch within 24 hours. "Any unexplained itch - think scabies"

SCARLET FEVER
"Streptococcal Toxic Erythema"

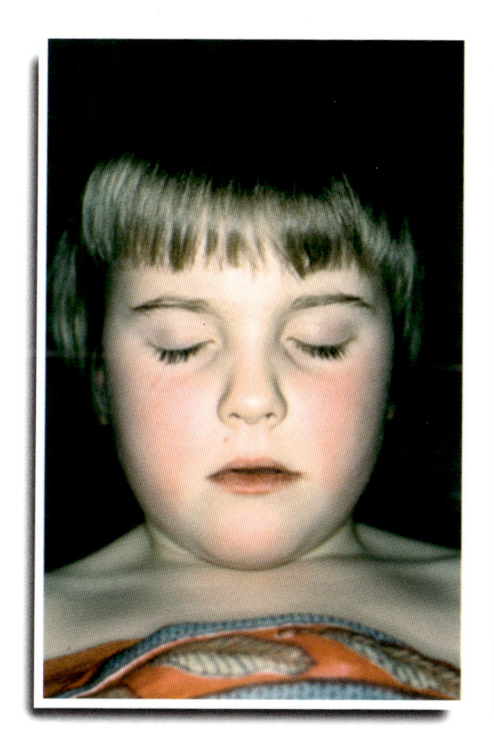

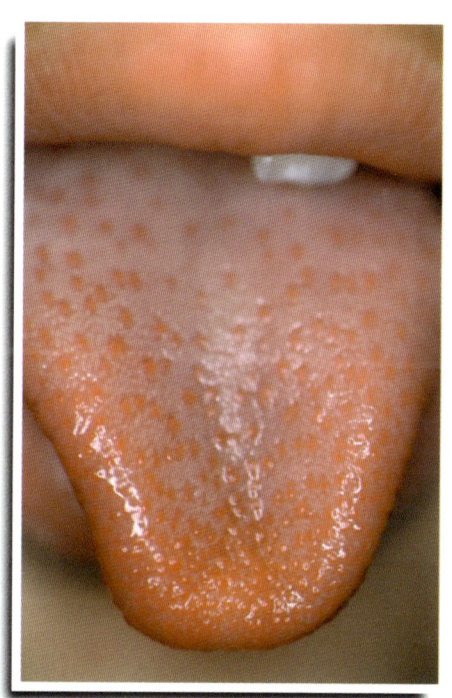

- Less common childhood infection (4 - 8 years) due Strep' Pyogenes + its' erythrogenic toxic
- Incubation 2 - 5 days. Sudden fever / anorexia / sore throat / exudative tonsillitis / lymphadenopathy
- Day 1 - furred tongue → red with prominent papillae = strawberry tongue
- Day 2 - widespread punctate erythema → confluent rash, skin can feel rough
- Classic signs: flushed face + circumoral pallor. Linear petechiae in axillae + groins (Pastia's lines)
- After 1 week, rash fades → peeling of palms and soles
- Complications: glomerulonephritis, erythema nodosum, myocarditis + rheumatic fever (↑ incidence)
- Treatment: oral Penicillin / Erythromycin + supportive measures

quick reference atlas of dermatology

SEBACEOUS CYST
"Epidermoid Cyst / Wen"

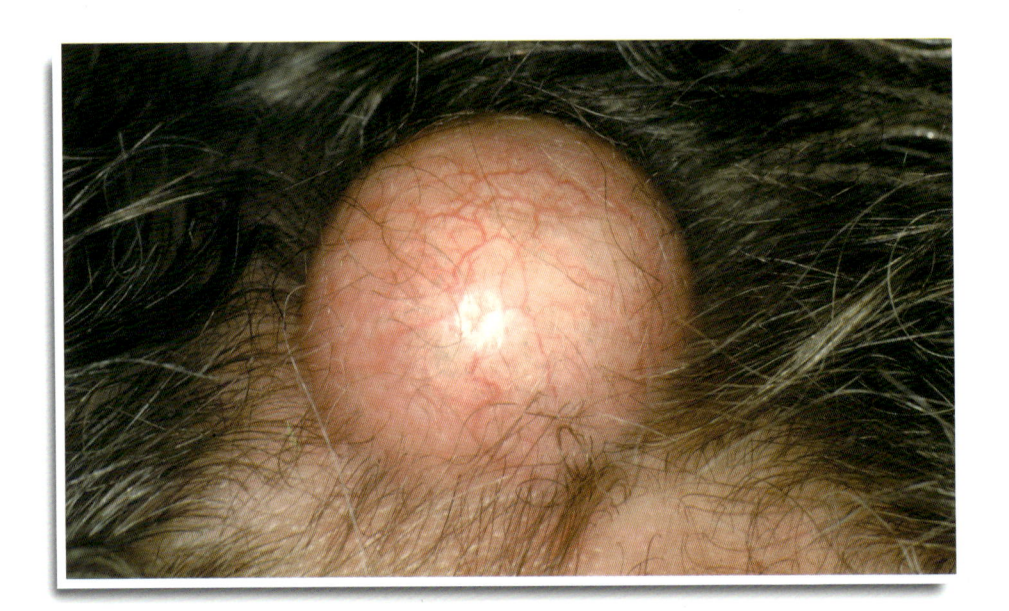

- Most common cutaneous cyst of primarily scalp, face, neck, shoulders, chest + scrotum in adults
- Well defined mobile papule / nodule within dermis, often with visible punctum
- Lining is normal epidermis from hair follicle sheath or sweat duct
- Offensive contents = lipid rich debris + altered keratin from epidermal lining
- Can also be an inherited autosomal dominant condition - appears after puberty
- If before puberty - associated with polyposis coli (Gardner's syndrome)
- Can occur after penetrating injury or acne damage to hair follicles
- Complications: secondary infection via punctum or rupture → tender inflammatory mass
- Treatment: cold excision with removal of entire cyst wall to prevent recurrence

SEBACEOUS HORN
"Cutaneous Horn"

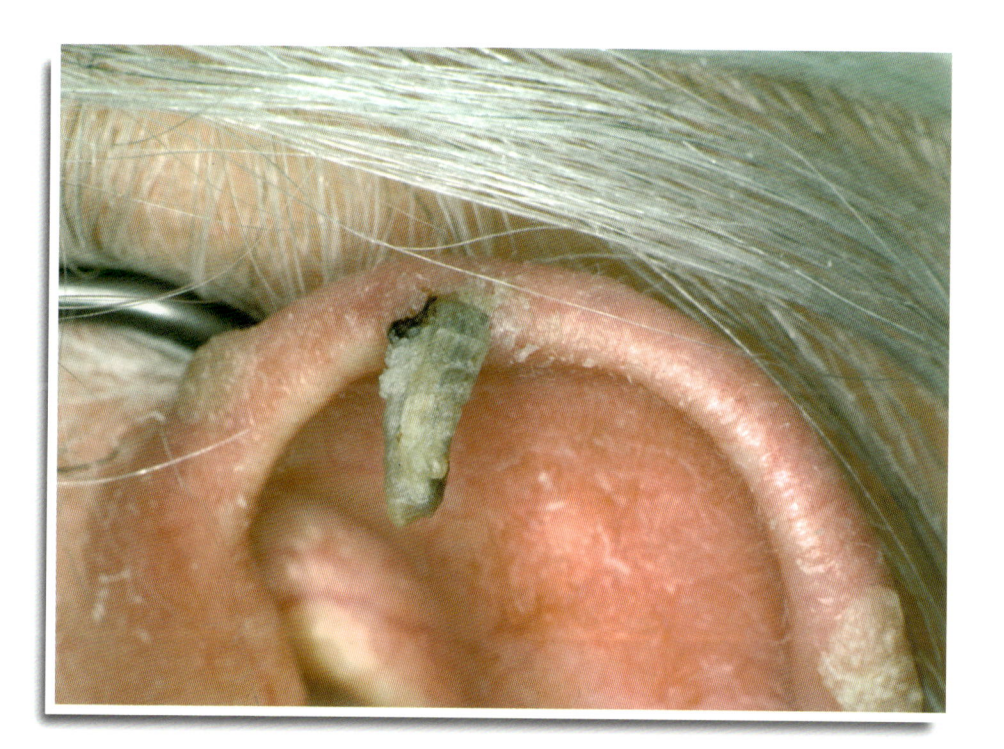

- Horny outgrowth usually overlying solar keratosis / Bowen's disease / SCC
- Solar keratoses more common in blue eyed fair skinned (especially Celts)
- Tend to arise on exposed areas e.g. face, ears, arms + hands
- Treatment: excise → histology to exclude SCC at base

SEBORRHOEIC WART
"Seborrhoeic Keratosis / Basal Cell Papilloma"

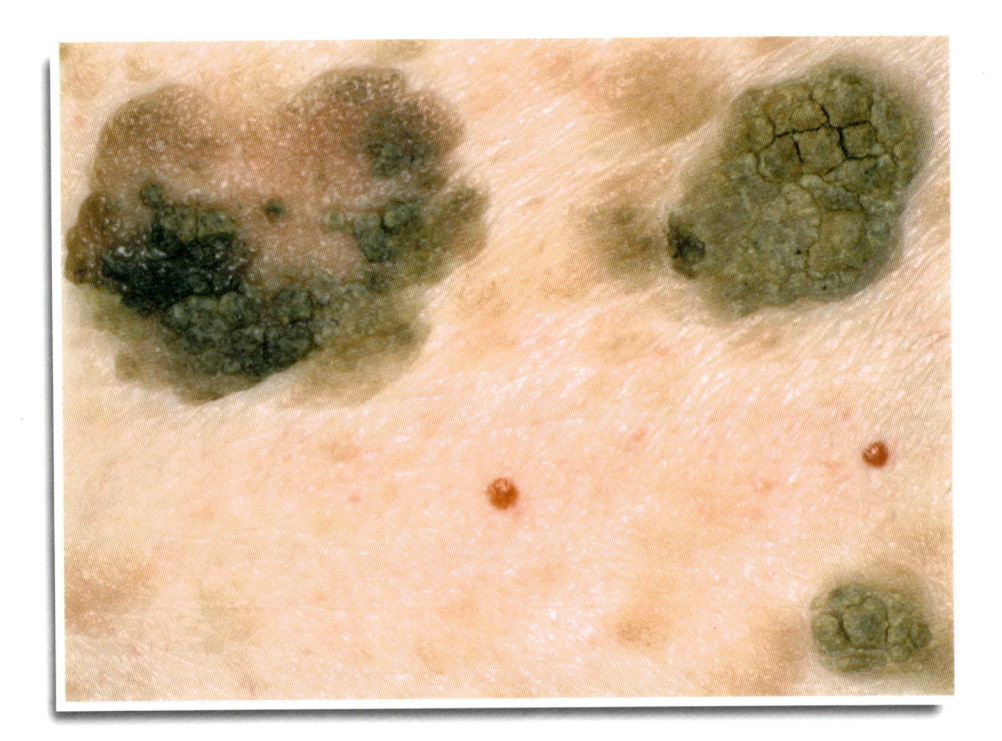

- Benign epidermal tumour not related to sebaceous glands
- Various size / colour (uniform) / shape. 0.5 - 3 cm diameter macule → papule / plaque
- Well defined edge + warty surface often with keratin plugs
- Stuck on appearance - like a "cow pat" or "Barnacles on the ship of life"
- Primarily > 40 years, Male > Female, often more extensive in men, ↑ incidence with age
- Solitary (face + neck) or multiple + large (trunk). Protuberant / pedunculated lesions can occur
- Causes: usually idiopathic or following inflammatory dermatosis
- Multiple lesions can be seen as autosomal dominant condition
- Sudden appearance of hundreds - seek internal neoplasm (Leser-Trelat's sign)
- Treatment: biopsy if in doubt, cryotherapy, cautery or curettage → histology

SKIN TAG
"Cutaneous Papilloma / Acrochordon"

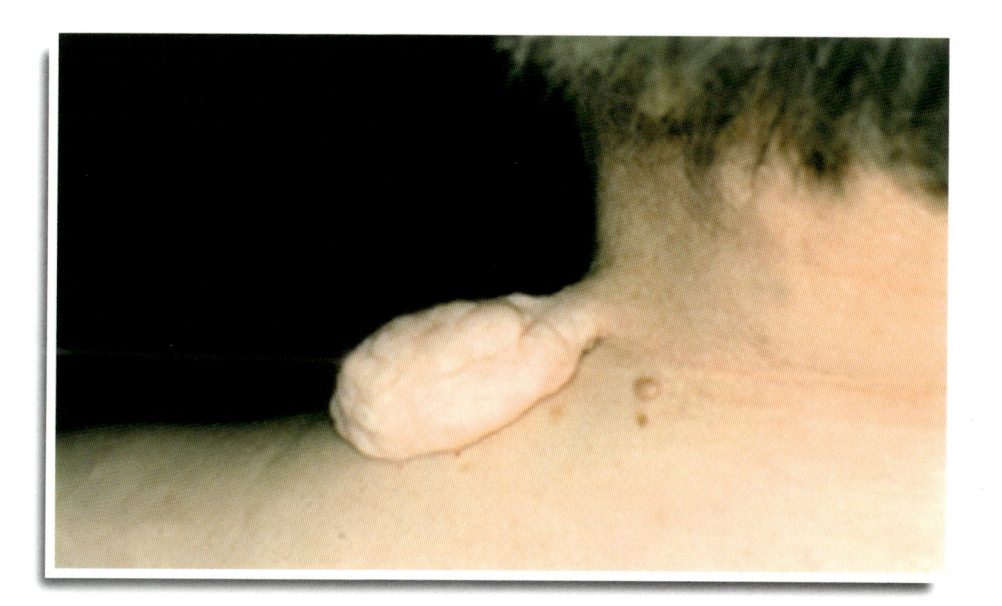

- Very common, benign, soft, skin / pink coloured pedunculated polyp
- Usually 1 - 10 mm diameter, constricted at its' base. Thin epidermis + fibrous stroma
- Sites: axillae, groin, neck, eyelids, inframammary area
- Primarily middle age → elderly, Female > Male, sometimes familial,
- Correlation with obesity + colonic polyps. ↑ number + size with time
- Easily traumatised → bleeding / crusting + possible autoamputation
- Rare association with: tuberose sclerosis, acanthosis nigricans, acromegaly + diabetes
- Treatment: if small can be snipped with scissors
- Usually excision with electrocautery or cryotherapy

SOLAR KERATOSES
"Actinic Keratoses / Sun Warts"

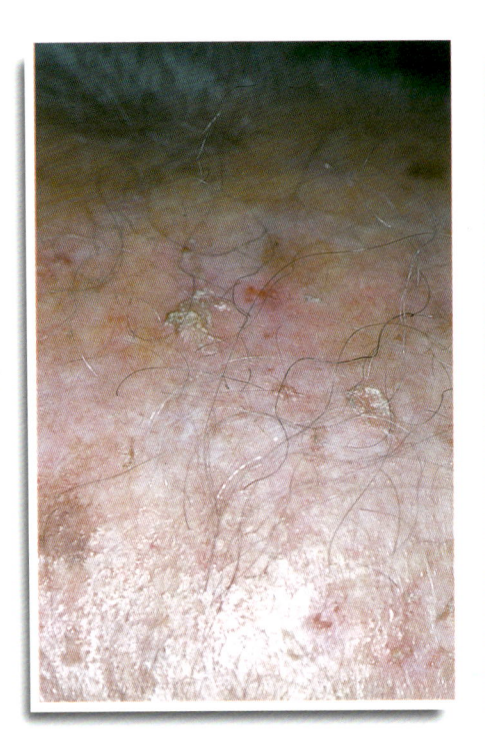

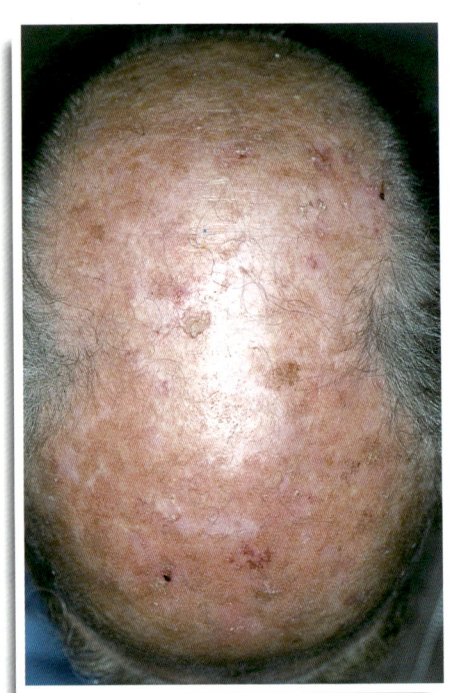

- Discrete, rough, adherent, scaly lesions with irregular periphery + surface
- Arise on sun exposed adult skin on background dermatoheliosis / photo aged skin
- Single or multiple lesions. Male = Female, middle age → elderly (<30 years in Australia + SW USA)
- Predisposing factors: excessive / protracted sun exposure, fair skin (· melanin is protective)
- Lesions are skin coloured / yellow / brown with reddish tinge, usually < 1 cm, oval / round
- Prime sites: face / ears / neck / forearms / hands / shins
- Gently scratching lesions → pain (a helpful diagnostic tool)
- Can disappear / persist for years or → nodular → malignant change (1 SCC from 1000 solar keratoses)
- Treatment: High SPF sun screen
- Cryotherapy → topical 5% 5-fluorouracil cream 3 days later to avoid depigmentation
- Curette larger lesions, biopsy if in doubt, excise nodular lesions.

SPIDER NAEVUS
"Spider Angioma / Naevus Araneus"

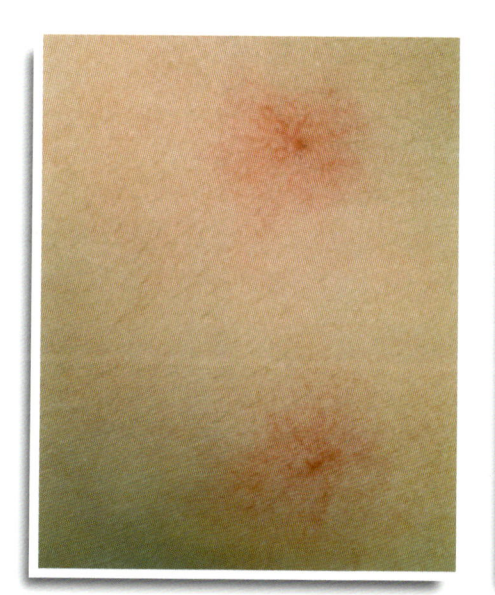

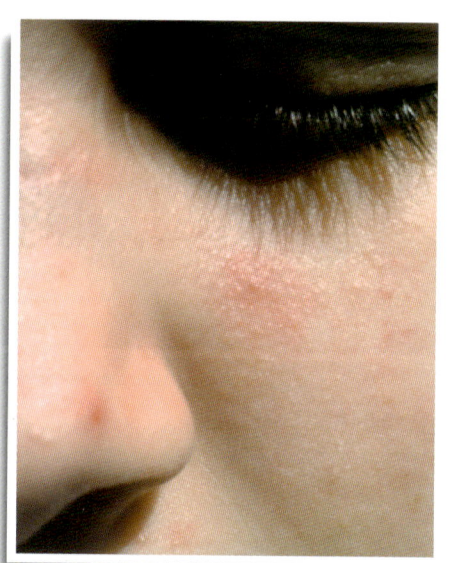

- Red, focal, telangiectatic network of dilated capillaries radiating from central arteriole
- Up to 1.5 cm diameter, solitary or multiple, primarily upper body, blanches with pressure
- Female >> Male, can occur in children age 2 - 6 years - often just under eye / cheek
- Associated with: ↑ oestrogen levels e.g. pregnancy / oral contraception + liver disease
- Can regress spontaneously (as in pregnancy + after puberty)
- Treatment: cold point cautery, hyfrecater or laser
- NB Salmon Patch = localised capillary, telangiectatic naevus found in new-born - no treatment required

SQUAMOUS CELL CARCINOMA
"SCC"

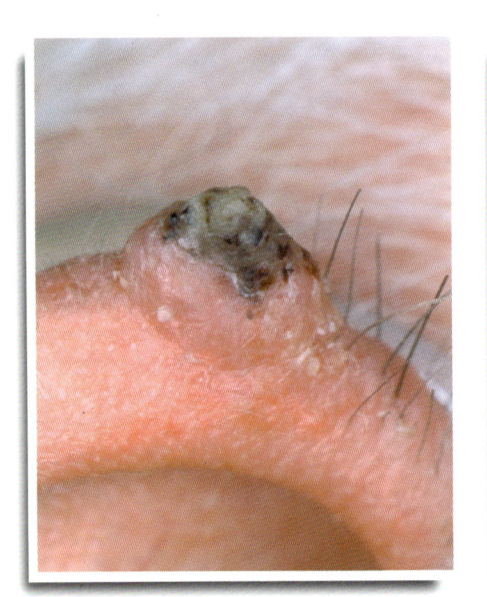

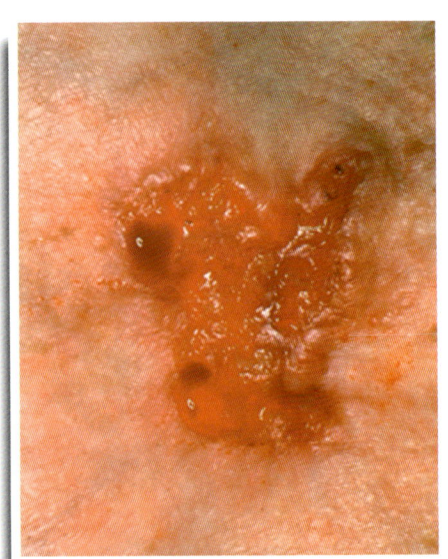

- Malignant tumour of skin + mucous membrane, less common than BCC
- Male > Female usually over 55 years (20 -30 in Australia)
- Occurs at sites with high solar damage - bald head, ears, dorsum hands, face, nose, lower lip
- Fast growing, craggy, indurated edge, elevated margin, ulcerates, crusted, bleeds easily
- Locally destructive, 3-4% metastasise, widespread metastases - untreatable
- 0.1% of solar keratoses undergo change to SCC
- If on unexposed areas, causes: arsenic, post radiation, burn scars, leg ulcers (frequently metastasise)
- Highly differentiated: keratinised + firm on palpation → curettage + cautery
- Poorly differentiated: fleshy, granulomatous + soft on palpation
- Treatment: Local excision + radiotherapy → 90% remission
- Very offensive large ulcerated lesions: excise + skin graft + block dissection of nodes

TINEA - CORPORIS
"Ringworm"

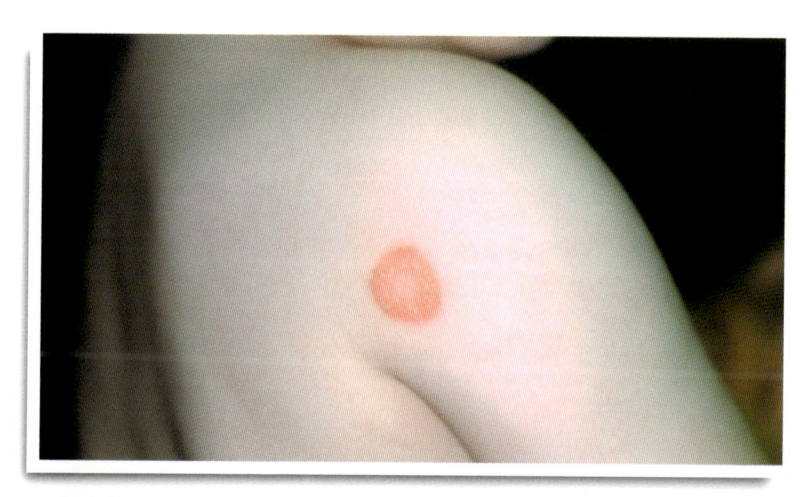

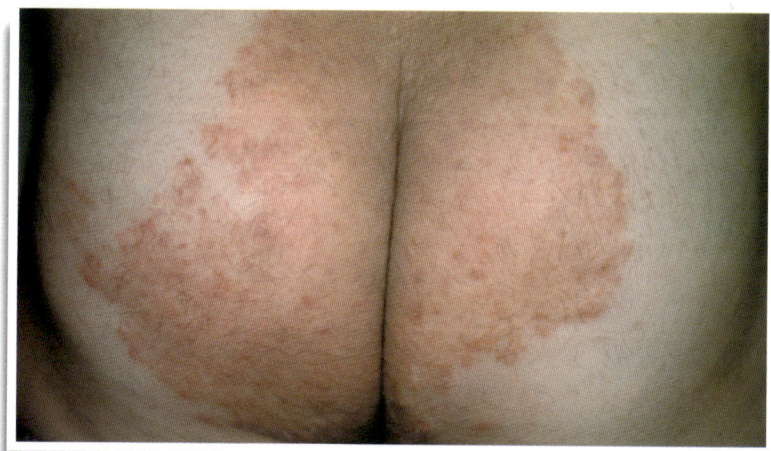

- Single or multiple, asymmetrical, red, scaly rash due to dermatophyte fungi invasion of keratin
- Microsporon (skin + hair), Trichophyton (skin, hair + nails) Epidermophyton (skin + nails)
- Well defined, pink, inflamed plaque spreads outwards → unused stratum corneum → central clearing
- Border of marked scaling / papules. Surrounding skin is normal
- Lesions on trunk + limbs, all ages, spread by autoinoculation, incubation days - months
- Worse inflammation if fungi from animals. Can be secondary to tinea capitis in children
- Treatment: examine skin scales from edge of lesion, topical or systemic antifungals for 2 - 4 weeks

TINEA - INCOGNITA

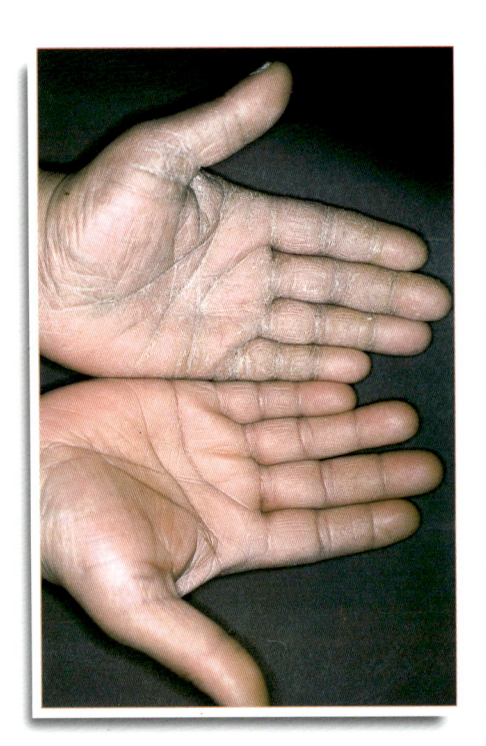

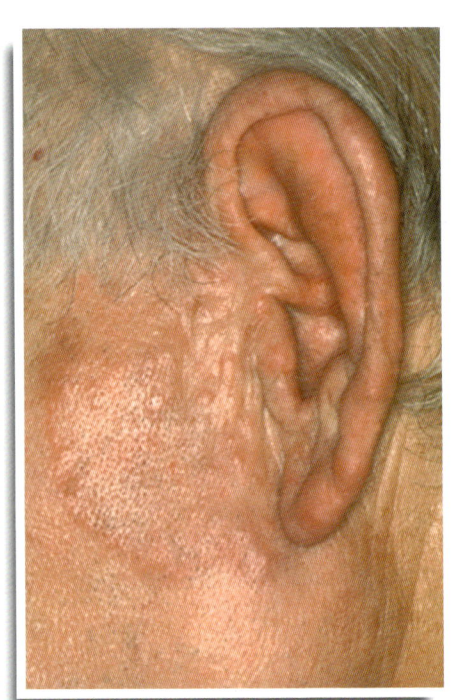

- Misdiagnosis of tinea → inappropriate steroid use → change in typical appearance
- Centre of ring more uniformly inflamed, less scaly, margins less well defined + pustular folliculitis
- Infecting organism flourishes → lesions persist and enlarge
- Primary sites groin / hand / face
- Treatment: stop steroids + use antifungals until cleared
- TINEA MANUUM - chronic dermatophyte infection of hands, usually unilateral on dominant side
- Usually associated with Tinea Pedis + Tinea Cruris,
- Can be mistaken for contact dermatitis + incorrectly treated with steroids → Tinea Incognita

TINEA - PEDIS
"Athlete's Foot"

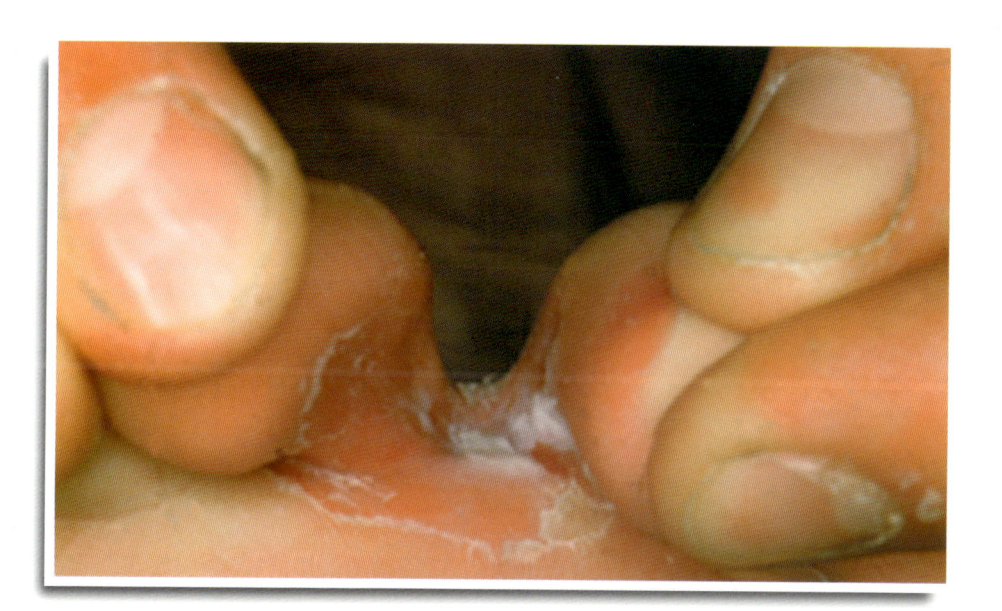

- Commonest fungal infection in man, very irritant, primarily 20 - 50 year olds, Male > Female
- 1. Commonest presentation: scaling of 4/5th inter-digital spaces, often unilateral, spreads medially → other foot → toe nails
- 2. "Moccasin type": scaly plaque extends from toe webs → dorsum of foot
- 3. Unilateral eruption of vesicles on instep. Fungus in roof of blisters, can ulcerate
- 4. White scaling of skin creases of sole of one / both feet, associated discolouration / thickening of toe nails (due to Trichophyton Rubrum)
- Can spread to hands due to scratching - "right hand / left foot" if right handed
- Secondary infection → maceration + offensive odour (diabetics + "vein harvesting leg" of CABG)
- Treatment: avoid occlusive footwear / persistent wearing same shoes / trainers
- Reduce sweating + humidity with cotton / wool socks
- Topical antifungals until two weeks after clearance, oral antifungals if recurrent / extensive / moccasin

URTICARIA
"Hives"

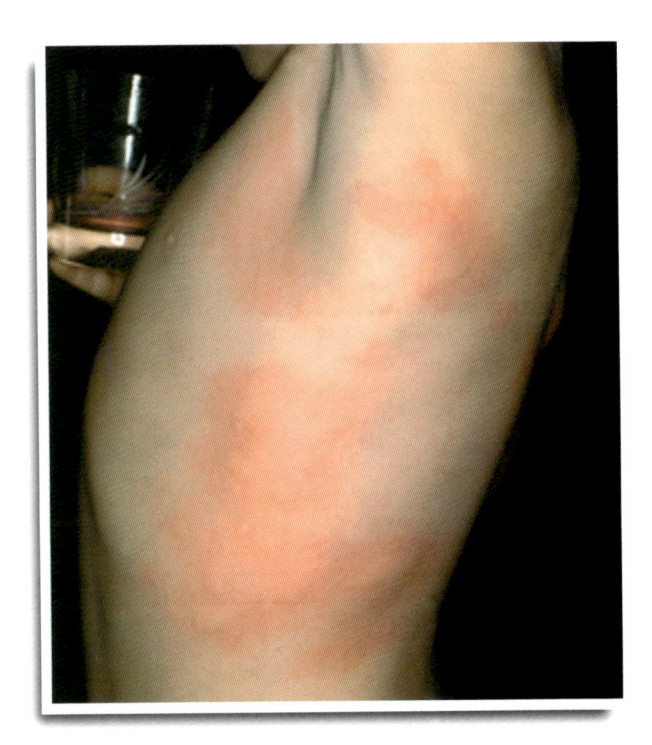

- A rash where lesions come + go within hours. Affects 15 - 20% population at some time
- Central, itchy white papule (due to dermal oedema) + erythematous flare = weal
- Lesions vary is size / shape. Mucosal involvement = angioedema
- Cause found in children > adults e.g. allergy, infection, physical stimuli
- ? due to histamine + other mediators released from skin mast cells
- Acute: lasts < 30 days. >70% of urticaria in children
- Type I (IgE mediated) allergic response within minutes of allergen contact (on skin or ingestion)
- Resolution within 1 hour. Often associated atopic background
- Chronic: lasts > 30 days. Primarily adults, Female : Male 2 : 1
- Comes + goes over months / years, lasts approximately 24 hours, new lesions keep appearing
- Causes: > 80% idiopathic, emotion / stress, food additives (Tartrazine), drugs: Aspirin / Codeine
- Also seen in association with hyperthyroidism, SLE, chronic active hepatitis
- Treatment: identify + avoid allergen if possible, none + reassurance, antihistamines, H2 blockers, Doxepin, tapering dose of oral steroids. If persistent → basic screening blood tests + examination

VARICOSE ULCERATION

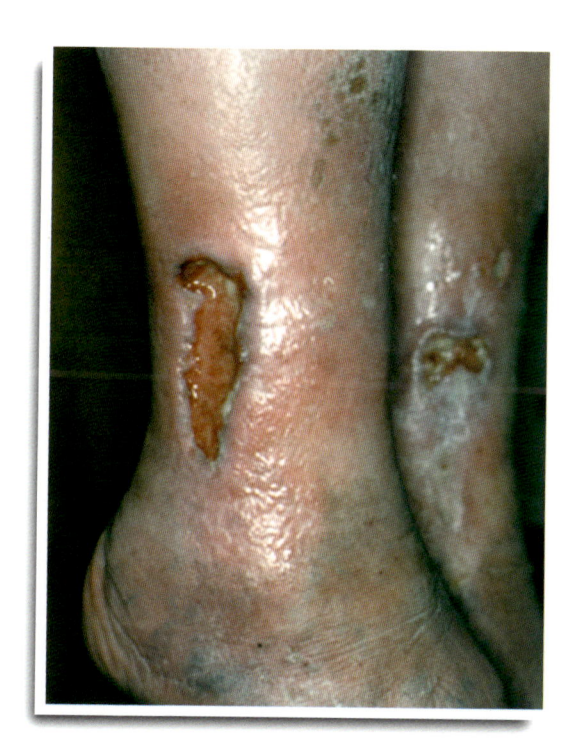

- 85 - 95% ulcers are venous / gravitational, primarily lower leg (malleolar area) involvement
- ↑ superficial vein / capillary pressure → oedema / purpura / venous flare + varicose veins → eczema → ulceration (due to reduced oxygen + nutrient supply)
- Female > Male, middle aged → elderly, normal pulses / sensation
- Obesity → increased + more severe ulceration, trivial trauma → ulcer in "compromised leg"
- Superficial, often large, painless ulcer with well defined, shelving edge + slough
- Complications: cellulitis / haemorrhage / soft tissue calcification / malignant change (Marjolin ulcer)
- Treatment: ideal → exudative phase → granulating phase → healing phase
- ↓ oedema, improve venous return, ↓ weight, ↑ exercise, remove slough, treat cellulitis
- Dressings, protect surrounding skin, maintain general health. Surgery (grafts + vascular)

VASCULITIS
"Allergic Angiitis / Necrotising Vasculitis"

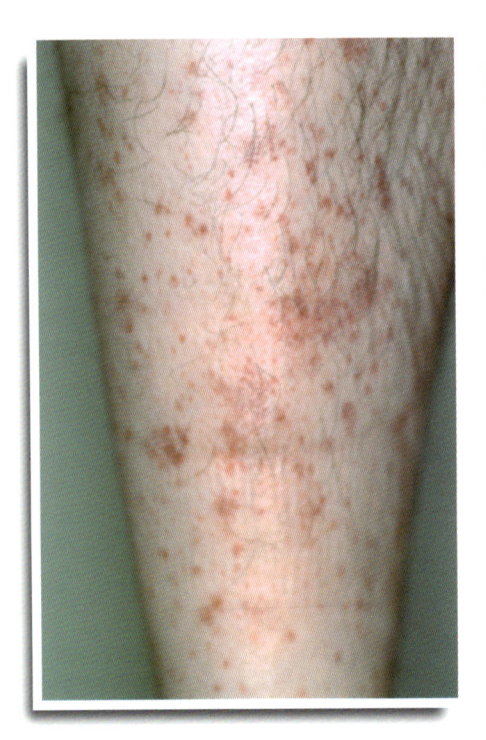

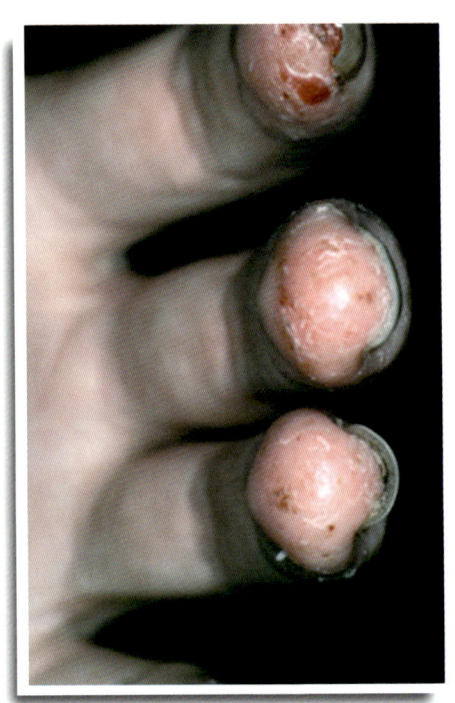

- Immune complex deposition in vein wall → inflammation, Male = Female 50% idiopathic
- Antigens: drugs (thiazides, antibiotics), infections (Strep', Hepatitis) + autoantigens (SLE, rheumatoid)
- Crops of lesions primarily on forearms / legs, pink → red macules / papules / vesicles
- Symptoms: none or possibly burning / itching
- Small vessel vasculitis: painful / palpable / purpura (PPP). Tissue over vessel can be necrotic
- Course varies according to cause / severity / size of vessels involved / other organ involvement
- Can be cutaneous or systemic. Organs involved: kidney, muscle, joints, GIT + peripheral nerves
- Can last days → years according to cause. If idiopathic can be recurrent over many years
- Treatment: treat cause, antihistamines + rest. If systemic: oral steroids +/- immunosuppressants

VERRUCAE
"Verrucae Plantaris / Plantar Warts"

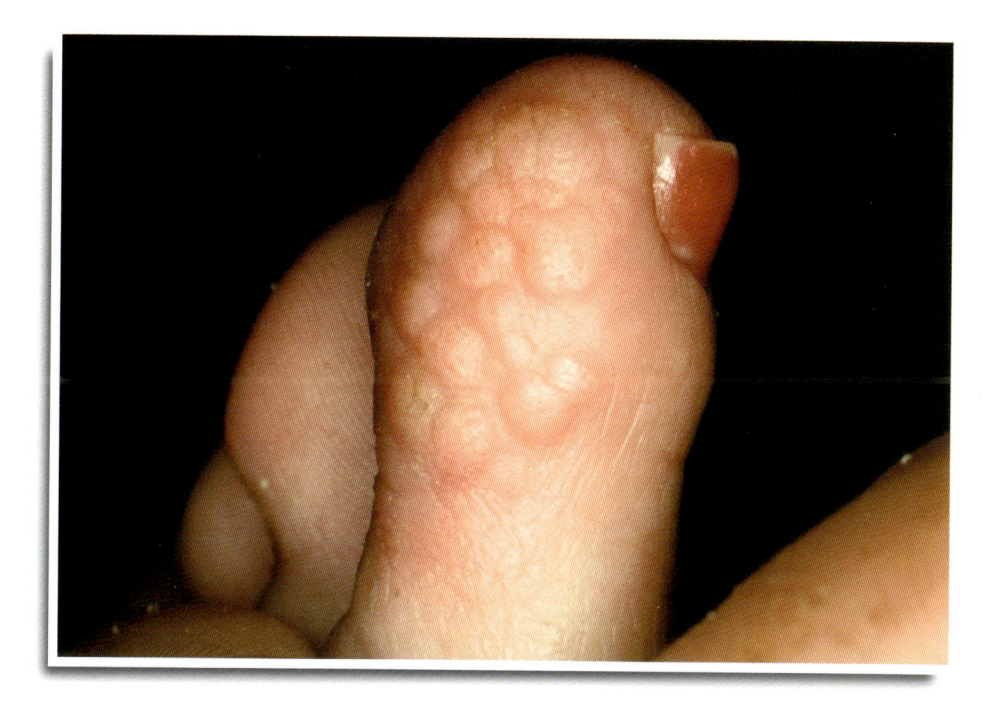

- 25% of all warts. Discrete round papules with rough surface + collar of hyperkeratosis
- Single or numerous confluent lesions (mosaic warts), aetiology - see VIRAL WARTS
- Paring surface with scalpel → tiny visible bleeding points
- Painful due to hyperkeratotic collar which acts like a stone in the shoe
- Thrombosis of vessels → severe pain → rapid resolution
- Treatment: preferably none - 70% resolve within 1 year, 90% within 2 years
- Very resistant to therapy as weight bearing drives the verruca deep into skin
- Pare down surface with scalpel / pumice stone → topical salicylic +/- lactic acid preparations
- Podophyllin + collodion flex preparations or as ointments
- Cryotherapy / electrocautery / curettage - at regular intervals
- N.B. "nature doesn't leave a scar so neither must you"

VIRAL WARTS
"Myrmecia"

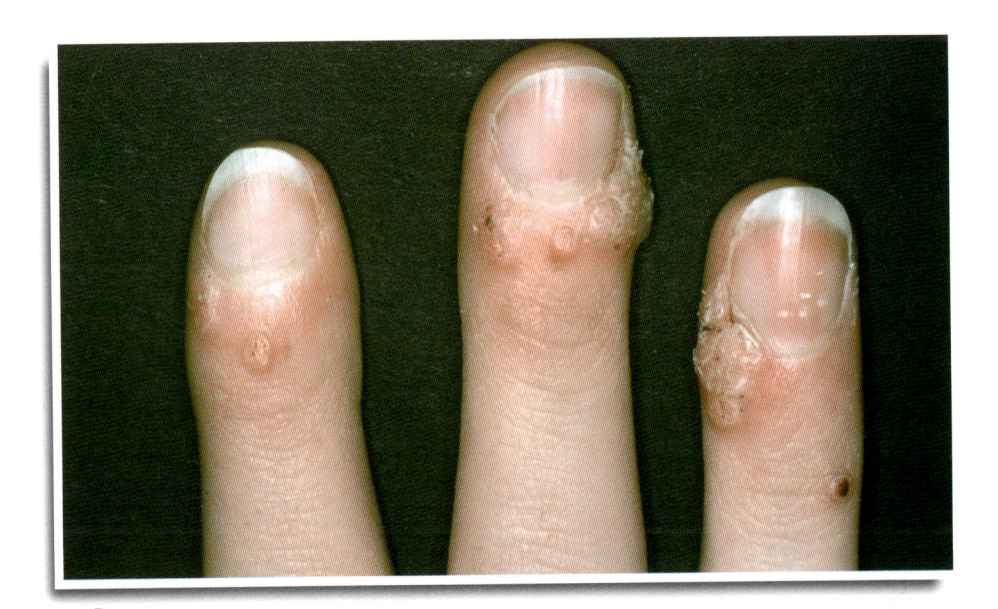

- Contagious, epidermal infection with one of approximately 50 human papilloma viruses
- Transmission via broken skin from one source to patient, trauma / nail biting → spread
- Spontaneous remission (2.5 years) due to cell mediated immune response
- Immunity to common wart virus does not prevent infection with verrucae or planar warts
- Common wart (verruca vulgaris) - 70% of all cutaneous warts. HPV 2, involves fingers + hand
- All ages, primarily 5 - 25 years. 1 - 10 mm firm, rough, skin coloured / brown papules
- Black dots on surface are visible thrombosed capillaries, normal skin lines are obscured
- Commonly occur around nails in children → depression of nail matrix → groove
- Extensive proliferation seen in immuno-suppressed conditions e.g. renal transplant
- Treatment: see verrucae, care with therapy as damage to nail matrix → permanent deformity

VIRAL WARTS - PLANAR

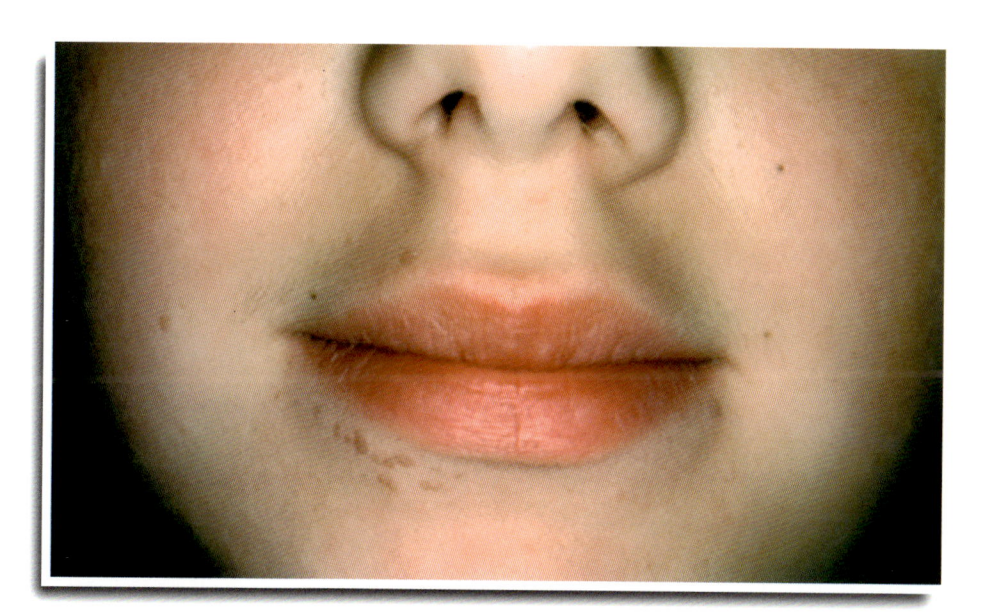

- Approximately 4% of all warts, small, flat topped, non-shiny papules
- Pink / brown + soft (not rough like common warts)
- Exhibit Koebner Phenomenon
- Primarily seen on dorsum of hands + face of children
- Treatment: rarely needed. If extensive → salicylic / lactic acid film preparations
- Cryotherapy may be helpful

VITILIGO

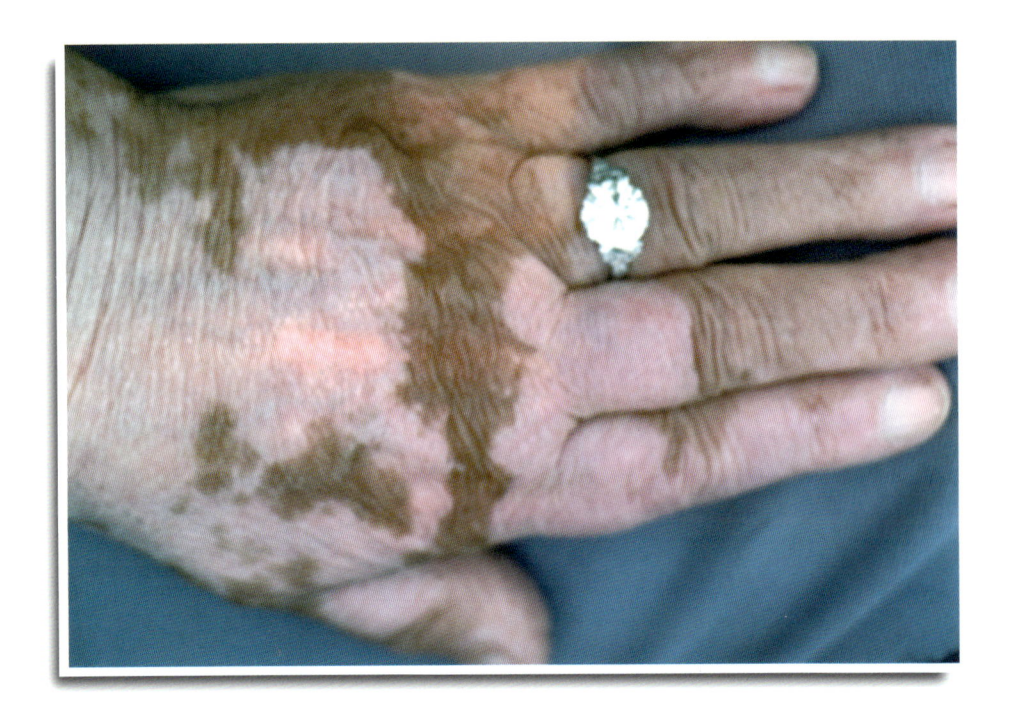

- Latin: vitellus = veal (pale pink flesh). Due to total loss of melanocytes
- Acquired depigmentation seen in all races, 0.5 - 1% prevalence, any age, Male = Female
- Trauma / sunburn are causative factors, lesions can demonstrate Koebner phenomenon
- Generalised (associated with autoimmune diseases) + segmental types
- Polygenic inheritance, 40% positive family history. No evidence it is an autoimmune condition in itself
- **Generalised:** appears after 2nd decade on backs of hands / wrist / knees / neck / around body orifices
- Hair of scalp + beard may depigment. In Caucasians adjacent skin may hyperpigment
- Lesions can remain static / spread / repigment spontaneously
- **Segmental**: striking localised distribution (in a band) on one side of body, often repigments
- Focal patches on a single site may proceed generalised + segmental variety
- Prognosis: best in patients with pigmented skin / minor lesions / isolated facial involvement
- Worst in Caucasians / extensive involvement / oral + finger / toe (Lip Tip syndrome)
- Treatment: unsatisfactory, best left alone + use high SPF sunscreens, cosmetic advice
- Short course potent topical steroids to recent patches, Psoralens + PUVA daily for 6 months
- Total / irreversible depigmentation using creams containing monobenzyl ether of hydroquinone

XANTHELASMA PALPEBRARUM
"Eyelid Xanthoma"

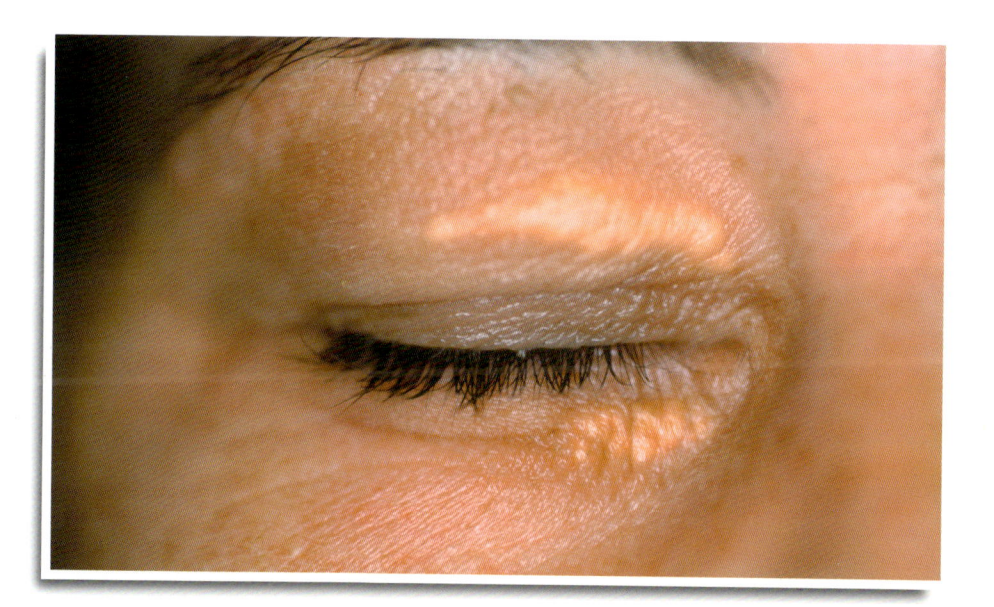

- Most common cutaneous xanthoma, primarily > 50 years old, Male = Female
- Yellow / brown, pink / orange slightly elevated plaques on or around eyelids
- May / may not be associated with hypercholesterolaemia (including dominantly inherited form)
- Histologically: macrophages containing lipid droplets
- Asymptomatic and enlarge slowly over months - years
- Treatment: treat high cholesterol (diet +/- lipid lowering agents), excision by plastic surgeon
- Electro-desiccation, laser, topical Trichloroacetic acid, recurrences uncommon

Index

A
ABSCESS,	4
ACANTHOSIS NIGRICANS,	5
ACNE ROSACEA,	6
ACNE VULGARIS,	7
Acrochordon,	103
Actinic Keratoses,	104
Adenoma Sebaceum,	43
Allergic Angiitis,	112
ALOPECIA AREATA,	9
ALOPECIA TOTALIS,	10
Alopecia Universalis,	10
Anaphylactic Purpura,	54
Angioedema,	110
ANGIOMA - CHERRY,	12
ANGIO-OEDEMA,	11
Athlete's Foot,	109
Atopic Eczema,	40
Auspitz Phenomenon,	90

B
BASAL CELL CARCINOMA,	13
Basal Cell Papilloma,	102
Bathing Trunk Naevus,	78
BCC,	13, 79
BECKER'S NAEVUS,	14
Blackhead,	7
BLACKHEADS,	15
BLUE NAEVUS,	16
Bowen's Disease,	101
BOWEN'S DISEASE,	17
Breslow's Thickness,	70
Bullae,	85, 89

C
CAFÉ AU LAIT,	18
Calcifying Epithelioma,	27
Campbell De Morgan Spot,	12
Candida,	82
CANDIDA,	19
CANDIDA - ORAL,	20
CAPILLARY HAEMANGIOMA,	21
CARBUNCLE,	22
CELLULITIS,	23
Chagrin Patches,	43
CHICKENPOX,	24, 57
CHLOASMA,	25
Clark Melanocytic Naevus,	37
Cold Sores,	55
Comedones,	15
Common Wart,	114
Compound Melanocytic Naevus,	77
Compound Naevus,	74, 77
Congenital Melanocytic Naevus,	78
Contact Dermatitis,	29
CRADLE CAP,	26
CUTANEOUS HORN,	101
Cutaneous Papilloma,	103
Cutaneous Xanthoma,	117
CYST OF MALHERBE,	27
Cystic Acne,	8

D
Dandruff,	32
DERMATITIS - ARTEFACTA,	28
DERMATITIS - CONTACT,	29
DERMATITIS - LIP LICKING,	30
DERMATITIS - PERIORAL,	31
DERMATITIS - SEBORRHOEIC,	32
DERMATOFIBROMA,	33
DERMATOGRAPHISM,	35
Dermatoheliosis,	104
DERMATOMYOSITIS - JUVENILE,	34
Discoid Eczema,	41
DRUG REACTIONS,	36
Dyshidrotic Eczema,	89
DYSPLASTIC NAEVUS SYNDROME,	37

E
Ecthyma,	59
ECTHYMA CONTAGIOSUM,	38
ECZEMA - ATOPIC,	39, 40
ECZEMA - DISCOID,	41
ECZEMA - VARICOSE,	42
Eczema Herpeticum,	62
Epidermal Naevus Syndrome,	79
Epidermoid Cyst,	100
EPILOIA,	43
ERYSIPELAS,	44
ERYTHEMA AB IGNE,	45
Erythema Induratum,	48
ERYTHEMA INFANTUM,	46
ERYTHEMA MULTIFORME,	47
ERYTHEMA NODOSUM,	48
Erythrasma,	107
Exanthem Subitum,	96
Exogenous Dermatitis,	29
Eyelid Xanthoma,	117

F
Fifth Disease,	46
Fitzpatrick's Sign,	33
FLEA BITES,	49
Folliculitis,	22
Furuncles,	22

G
Gardner's Syndrome,	100
German Measles,	97
Gottron's Papules,	34
GRANULOMA ANNULARE,	50, 81
Granuloma Telangiectaticum,	95
Gravitational Eczema,	42
GUTTATE PSORIASIS,	51

H
HALO NAEVUS,	52
HAND, FOOT + MOUTH,	53
HENOCH SCHONLEIN PURPURA,	54
Herald Patch,	87
Herpes Simplex,	47, 62
HERPES SIMPLEX LABIALIS,	55
HERPES ZOSTER,	57, 24
HERPETIC WHITLOW,	56
Histiocytoma,	33
Hives,	110
Housewife's Dermatitis,	29
Hutchinson's Freckle,	70

I
Ichthyosis,	39
ICHTHYOSIS VULGARIS,	58, 65
IMPETIGO,	59
INSECT BITES,	60
Intradermal Naevus,	74, 77
Intraepidermal Epithelioma,	17

J
Jadassohn's Phakomatosis,	79
Jock Itch,	107
Junctional Naevus,	74, 77
JUVENILE PLANTAR DERMATOSIS,	61

K
KAPOSI'S VARICELLIFORM ERUPTION,	62
KELOID,	63
Keratin Cysts,	73
KERATOACANTHOMA,	64
KERATOSIS PILARIS,	65, 39, 58
Koebner Phenomenon,	66, 90, 115
Koenen's Tumours,	43
Koplik's Spots,	68

L
Langer's Lines,	87
Leser-Trelat's Sign,	102

118 quick reference atlas of dermatology

Index

LICHEN PLANUS,	66
LICHEN SIMPLEX CHRONICUS,	67
Linea Nigra,	25
Lip Licking Dermatitis,	30
Lip Tip Syndrome,	116

M

Malignant Melanoma,	52, 80
Marjolin Ulcer,	111
MEASLES,	68
Melanocytic Naevus,	74, 78
MELANOMA,	69
Melasma,	25
MENINGOCOCCAL RASH,	71
METASTATIC NODULES,	72
MILIA,	73
MOLE,	74
MOLLUSCUM CONTAGIOSUM,	75
MONGOLIAN BLUE SPOT,	76
Moniliasis,	19
Mosaic Warts,	113
Myrmecia,	1, 14

N

NAEVUS - COMPOUND MELANOCYTIC,	77
NAEVUS - CONGENITAL MELANOCYTIC,	78
NAEVUS - SEBACEOUS,	79
NAEVUS - SPILUS,	80
Naevus - Strawberry,	21
Naevus Araneus,	105
Napkin Dermatitis,	19
Napkin Psoriasis,	90
NECROBIOSIS LIPOIDICA,	81
Necrotising Vasculitis,	112
Neurofibromatosis,	18, 80
Nikolsky Sign,	86
Nummular Eczema,	41

O

Onycholysis,	82
ONYCHOMYCOSIS,	82
Orf,	38
Organoid Naevus,	79

P

PALMAR ERYTHEMA,	83
Papillomatous Hamartoma,	79
PARONYCHIA,	84, 82
Pastia's Lines,	99
PEMPHIGOID - BULLOUS,	85
PEMPHIGUS VULGARIS,	86
Perioral Dermatitis,	31

Pilomatrixoma,	27
Pityriasis Amantacea,	93
PITYRIASIS ROSEA,	87
PITYRIASIS VERSICOLOR,	88
Plantar Warts,	113
POMPHOLYX,	89
PSORIASIS - FLEXURAL,	91
PSORIASIS - PLAQUE,	90
PSORIASIS - PUSTULAR,	92
PSORIASIS - SCALP,	93
Psoriasis Guttate,	51
Pustular Dermatitis,	38
PYODERMA GANGRENOSUM,	94
PYOGENIC GRANULOMA,	95

R

Reye's Syndrome,	24
Ringworm,	107
Rodent Ulcer,	13
ROSEOLA INFANTUM,	96
RUBELLA,	97

S

Salmon Patch,	106
SCABIES,	98
SCARLET FEVER,	99
SCC,	17, 64, 101, 104, 106
SEBACEOUS CYST,	100
SEBACEOUS HORN,	101
Sebaceous Naevus,	79
Sebaceous Naevus Of Jadassohn,	79
Seborrhoeic Dermatitis,	26, 32
Seborrhoeic Keratosis,	102
SEBORRHOEIC WART,	102
Shingles,	57
SKIN TAG,	103
SOLAR KERATOSES,	104, 101, 106
Spider Angioma,	105
Spider Naevus,	83
SPIDER NAEVUS,	105
Spilus Naevus,	80
SQUAMOUS CELL CARCINOMA,	106
Stasis Eczema,	42
Steven Johnson Syndrome,	47
Strawberry Naevus,	21
Streptococcal Toxic Erythema,	99
Sun Warts,	104
Sutton's Naevus,	52

T

Three Day Measles,	97
TINEA - CORPORIS,	107
Tinea Cruris,	107, 108

TINEA - INCOGNITA,	108
Tinea Manuum,	108
TINEA - PEDIS,	109, 108
Tinea Unguium,	84
Tinker's Tartan,	45
Toxic Sock Syndrome,	61
Tuberose Sclerosis,	43

U

URTICARIA,	110, 11

V

Varicella Zoster,	24
Varicose Eczema,	42
VARICOSE ULCERATION,	111
VASCULITIS,	112
Verruca Vulgaris,	114
VERRUCAE,	113
Verrucae Plantaris,	113
Vesicular Palmar Eczema,	89
VIRAL WARTS,	113, 114
VIRAL WARTS - PLANAR,	115
VITILIGO,	116, 52
Von Recklinghausen's Disease,	18
Von Zumbusch's Disease,	92

W

WARTS,	114
Wen,	100
Whitehead,	7, 15
Wickham's Striae,	66

X

XANTHELASMA PALBEBRARUM,	117
Xerosis,	39

quick reference atlas of dermatology

119

Bibliography

Ankrett VO. & Williams I.
Atlas Casebook of Primary Care.
Merit International.

Ashton R. & Leppard B.
Differential Diagnosis in Dermatology.
Radcliffe.

Ashton R. & Leppard B.
Treatment in Dermatology.
Radcliffe.

Buxton PK.
ABC of Dermatology.
BMJ.

Fitzpatrick TB. et al.
Color Atlas and Synopsis of Clinical dermatology.
McGraw-Hill.

Higgins E. & du Vivier A.
Skin Diseases in Childhood and Adolescence.
Blackwell.

Hunter JAA. et al.
Clinical Dermatology.
Blackwell.

Marks R.
Practical Problems in Dermatology.
Martin Dunitz.

Verbov J. & Morley N.
Colour Atlas of Paediatric Dermatology.
MTP Press.

White G.
Levene's Colour Atlas of Dermatology.
Mosby-Wolfe.